Religious Therapeutics

SUNY series in Religious Studies

Harold Coward, editor

Religious Therapeutics

Body and Health
in Yoga, Āyurveda, and Tantra

GREGORY P. FIELDS

STATE UNIVERSITY OF NEW YORK

Published by
State University of New York Press, Albany

Printed in the United States of America

For information, address State University of New York Press,
90 State Street, Suite 700, Albany, N.Y. 12207

Production, Laurie Searl
Marketing, Dana E. Yanulavich

Library of Congress Cataloging-in-Publication Data

Fields, Gregory P., 1961–
Religious therapeutics : body and health in yoga, Ayurveda, and Tantra/Gregory P. Fields.
p. cm. — (SUNY series in religious studies)
Includes bibliographical references and index.
ISBN 0-7914-4915-7 (alk. paper) — ISBN 0-7914-4916-5 (pbk. : alk. paper)
1. Medicine, Ayurvedic. 2. Medicine—Religious aspects—Hinduism. 3. Yoga.
4. Tantrism. 5. Body, Human— Religious aspects—Hinduism. I. Title. II. Series.
R606.F53 2001
615.5'3—dc21 00-049234

10 9 8 7 6 5 4 3 2 1

Contents

Chapter Four
TANTRA AND AESTHETIC THERAPEUTICS   139

Conclusion
COMMUNITY:
RELATIONALITY IN RELIGIOUS THERAPEUTICS   167

Figures

Tables

ACKNOWLEDGMENTS

Thanks first to K. N. Upadhyaya, Emeritus Professor of Philosophy, University of Hawaii. Also of the Department of Philosophy at the University of Hawaii, I thank Roger T. Ames, Eliot Deutsch, and Steve Odin. Special thanks to Cromwell Crawford, of the Department of Religion at the University of Hawaii. Thanks to Southern Illinois University at Edwardsville for two Summer Research Fellowships for travel to India and revision of the manuscript. Thanks to R. Neelameggham for contribution of the font for diacriticals, and to Hariharan Śrinivasan for technical assistance. Thanks to Harold Coward of the University of Victoria, editor of the *Series in Religious Studies*, and Nancy Ellegate and Laurie Searl of the State University of New York Press. Thanks to John Thomas Casey of the Department of Theological Studies at Loyola Marymount University for his drawing of Śri Yantra, and to Tammy Epperson for the cover concept. For generous help with the index, thanks to Katrina Lemke and Juli Jacobson. I am very thankful for the abundance and opportunities that allowed me to do this work. Great thanks to family and friends for countless instances of help, and to all those who have contributed in many ways to the completion of this book.

Symbols and Notes on Sources

Radical	√	indicates Sanskrit verbal roots or Indo-European root words.
Single brackets	[ ]	in translations enclose words added for clarification.

Quotations from the *Yoga-sūtras* are translated by Gregory P. Fields.

Quotations from the *Yoga-bhāṣya* and the *Tattva-vaiśāradī* are from the English translation *Patañjali's Yoga Sūtras* by Rāma Prasāda (New Delhi: Munshiram Manoharlal, 1912, 1978).

Quotations from the Āyurvedic text *Caraka-saṃhitā* and its commentary *Āyurveda-dīpikā* are from the translation of R. K. Sharma and Bhagwan Dash: *Caraka-saṃhitā of Agniveśa: Text with English Translation and Critical Exposition Based on Cakrapaṇidatta's Āyurveda Dīpikā*, 3 vols. (Varanasi: Chowkhamba Sanskrit Series, Vol. 94, 1976). Clarifications are provided based on the translation of P. V. Sharma: *Caraka-saṃhitā: Agniveśa's Treatise Refined and Annotated by Charaka and Redacted by Dṛḍhabala*, 4 vols. (Varanasi: Chaukhamba Orientalia, Jaikrishnadas Āyurveda Series, Vol. 36, 1994, 1995), in consultation with etymological and secondary sources.

Quotations from the Tāntric texts *Mahānirvāṇa Tantra* and *Ṣaṭcakra-nirūpaṇa* are from, respectively: *The Great Liberation* (Madras: Ganesh and Co., 1913, 1953), and *The Serpent Power* (Madras: Ganesh and Co., 1918, 1964), both translated by Arthur Avalon (Sir John Woodroffe).

Etymological analyses of Sanskrit terms are based on:

English-Sanskrit Dictionary by V. S. Apte. New Delhi: Publications India, reprint 1989.

A Practical Sanskrit Dictionary by Arthur Anthony Macdonnell. Oxford: Oxford University Press, 1924, 1990.

A Sanskrit-English Dictionary by Sir Monier Monier-Williams. Oxford: Oxford University Press, 1899, 1974.

The Roots, Verb-Forms and Primary Derivatives of the Sanskrit Language by William Dwight Whitney. New Haven, CT: American Oriental Society, 1885, 1945.

Secondary sources are cited in endnotes, and primary sources are cited in the body of the text, identified by the abbreviations on the next page.

Abbreviations

AV	*Atharva-veda*
AD	*Āyurveda-dīpikā*
BhG	*Bhagavadgītā*
CS	*Caraka-saṃhitā*
HYP	*Haṭha Yoga Pradīpikā*
MNT	*Mahānirvāṇa Tantra*
RV	*Ṛg-veda*
SK	*Sāṃkhya-kārikā*
SKB	*Sāṃkhya-kārikā-bhāṣya*
SCN	*Ṣaṭ-cakra-nirūpaṇa*
TV	*Tattva-vaiśāradī*
Up.	*Upaniṣads*
	Bṛhad. Up. *Bṛhadāraṇyaka*
	Chānd. Up. *Chāndogya*
	Kaṭh. Up. *Kaṭha*
	Mait. Up. *Maitri*
	Muṇḍ. Up. *Muṇḍaka*
	Śvet. Up. *Śvetāśvatara*
	Tait. Up. *Taittirīya*
VC	*Viveka-cūḍāmaṇi*
YBh	*Yoga-bhāṣya*
YS	*Yoga-sūtras*

Introduction

The Idea of Religious Therapeutics

World religious traditions abound with connections between healing and spirituality—for instance, the work of Jesus as savior and healer. Another example is Navajo religion's focus on healing as restoration of well-being to persons who suffer some form of digression from the flow of the life-force. The Hindu religio-philosophical tradition, operating from the premise that life is suffering, is a rich source of therapeutics to remedy the human condition. The Hindu subtraditions are in general concerned with well-being of persons in their spiritual dimension, and thus emerges a concept of 'spiritual health.' This study examines relations among body, health, and religiousness in Āyurveda, classical Yoga, and Tantra. These three traditions treat the relationship between embodied life and sacred life in ways that are interestingly different from standard Western views. And because of their emphasis on physicality, these three traditions are also unusual in the Hindu context, since Hinduism has a strong inclination to conceive of spiritual Self-realization or God-realization as entailing transcendence of physicality.

The idea of *religious therapeutics* embraces principles and practices that support human well-being with recognition of the common ground and cooperation of health and religiousness. Dimensions of religious therapeutics include the following:

Major Dimensions of Religious Therapeutics

- Religious meanings that inform philosophy of health and medicine
- Religious means of healing

- Health as a support to religious life
- Religiousness itself as a remedy for the suffering of the human condition

The idea of religious therapeutics can apply to any number of relations among health, healing, and religiousness. Taking a broad view, a whole tradition can be examined from the standpoint of its therapeutic impetus, or the term *religious therapeutic* can designate specific principles and practices, such as meditation, or use of prayer for healing.

In recent decades, there has been a surge of interest in health and healing in the context of spirituality. Humankind has an increasingly sharp awareness of threats to the health of the earth and its inhabitants, and of spiritual poverty as one of the factors underlying damage to environmental and human health. Contemporary thought and culture show strong interest in healing—physical, psychological, environmental, societal, political, and religious. The model of religious therapeutics is offered as a heuristic or interpretive lens for identifying and understanding relations among healing and religiousness in Hindu and other world traditions. Philosophically, the many constellations of factors in the common domain of religion and medicine reveal a great deal about the human being—embodied and spiritual. In addition, I hope that an evolving model of religious therapeutics will contribute to a more satisfactory account of health, applicable to human life in its many dimensions, including the spiritual, thus informing productive work in philosophy of medicine, health education, health-care, and health-related pastoral care.

RELIGION AND MEDICINE

Religion and medicine are distinct fields of human endeavor, but the need for well-being of body, mind, and spirit marks the common ground of medical and religious effort. The idea of religious therapeutics is evident is Paul Tillich's position on the intimate relation of religion and healing. His view is based on New Testament accounts of healing, which he says should not be taken as miracle stories, but as illustrations of Jesus' identity as the universal healer. Human beings in their finitude require 'particular' healing, that is, healing of specific ailments through surgical, pharmaceutical, psychotherapeutic, and like means. But the human being in his or her ultimate nature needs salvation or liberation in a total and ultimate sense. Jesus as healer embodies the meaning of savior: the (Gk.) *sōtēr* or healer is the one who makes healthy and whole.[1]

The idea of religious therapeutics demands inquiry into the relationship of soteriology (the theory of salvation) with health and healing. The common ground of salvation and healing is evident in etymological analysis. The words 'soteriology' and 'savior' are derived from the Greek verb *sōzein*, 'to save.'[2] The Latin equivalent is *salvāre*, which is the source of the word 'salvation.'[3] The Indo-European root √*sol-* (variant √*sal-*) means 'whole.' Descendents of √*sol-* include the Latin *sālus*, health or wholeness, and the English words *save* and *salvation.*[4] *Salvāre* can denote religious salvation, and can also mean 'to make whole.'[5] 'To make whole' is the literal meaning of the Old English verbal root *hāl*, origin of the word *heal*. *Heal* carries the meaning of *restoration* from an undesirable condition, and at an elemental level pertains to saving, purifying, cleansing, and repairing to bring about restoration from evil, suffering, or unwholesomeness. These are also functions of religion. Reference to *healing* in the domains of human physicality and psychology is the most common use of the word, but the fundamental meaning of *healing* is recovery of wholeness, which spiritual liberation entails.

The word *therapeutic* is from the Greek *therapúein*, and pertains to curing and restoring. The term *therapeía*, healing (akin to *therápōn*, 'attendant'), can connote religious or medical endeavor, for it refers to the attending of a healer to a patient, and also designates 'attending' in the form of religious ministering.[6] The terms 'cure' and 'restore' reveal two perspectives on healing. *Curing* refers to alleviating impaired functioning and discomfort, while *restoring* connotes returning to an original state of well-being. These two meanings support a conception of healing as having religious as well as medical implications. The close relationship between healing and religion is well substantiated in the Indian tradition, where liberation is often construed as return to the unimpaired state of one's true nature. This is reflected in the Sanskrit terms for health, *svāsthya* and *svasthatā*: 'self-abiding' or 'coinciding with oneself' (*sva* 'oneself'; √*sthā* 'to stand'). Wilhelm Halbfass notes in his analysis of the Indian tradition's therapeutic paradigms that in Advaita Vedānta, these two terms are used by Śaṅkara and his disciple Sureśvara "to refer to their soteriological goal, the unobstructed presence and identity of the *ātman*."[7] The comparable term in classical Yoga is *svarūpe 'vastānam*: establishment in one's own essential nature, which is Yoga's prime goal [YS 1.3].

Contemporary interest in religious therapeutics is evident in the expansion of research activity under the rubric of religion and medicine. For instance, in his article "Mantra in Āyurveda" Kenneth Zysk writes:

> At all times and in almost every culture, a connection between medicine and religion is demonstrable. The belief that by soliciting divine intervention through prayer and ritual no disease is incurable cuts across cultural boundaries.[8]

Zysk's emphasis here is medical applications of religious speech in Āyurveda, and although religious therapeutics may include religious means of treating health problems, religious therapeutics embrace many other relations between healing and religiousness. In classical Yoga, physical and psychological maladies may be remedied by religious effort, but such healing is instrumental to a more fundamental healing: restoration to one's Self-nature as consciousness, unencumbered by psychophysical limitations.

Religion and medicine serve the common purpose of helping persons with transitions through the stages of living and dying, and they share the aim of remedying human suffering. In India, the relation that obtains between religion and medicine is importantly different from that of the dominant tradition of the Anglo-European world, where science and religion are treated more dichotomously. In the West, medicine is oriented toward the body and life in the present world, while religion is considered the province of non-material spirit, and particularly concerned with an afterlife. In the Indian tradition, there is a much greater affinity between religion and medicine. One of the major commentaries on the *Yoga-sūtras*, Vācaspati-miśra's *Tattva-Vaiśāradī*, states that the science of Yoga is similar to the science of medicine for both "are taught for the welfare of all" [TV 2.15]. The contrast of Anglo-European and Indian perspectives on religion and medicine is rooted in their divergent metaphysical conceptions of person, body, and human potential. The Indian tradition has a more holistic view of the human being as a unity, with psychophysical and spiritual dimensions. The first three of the traditional four aims of life (*dharma*, righteousness; *artha*, material well-being; *kāma*, enjoyment; and *mokṣa*, liberation) serve embodied well-being, but, more than that, each can contribute to attainment of the fourth and ultimate goal: self-realization and spiritual liberation.

Anglo-European and Indian approaches to health and spirituality diverge also in the way the two traditions regard knowledge. While the Indian tradition in general gives more credence to intuitive and mystical knowledge, in the West, science and reason are strongly valued. Medicine in the Anglo-European tradition relies heavily on empirical knowledge, but in Hinduism, religious knowledge, and, to a large extent, medical knowledge, are rooted in the Vedic knowledge intuited by ancient seers. Vedic knowledge is considered to provide comprehension that is more complete and truthful than knowledge gained through the senses. Āyurveda exemplifies cooperation of empirical and intuitive knowledge, and attention to both earthly and spiritual concerns.

From the standpoint of value theory, the Western presupposition that rationality is among the highest goods supports the application of reason and knowledge for utilization of the earth's natural resources. Technologically developed material resources are central to diagnosis and treatment in contemporary scientific medicine, evident in the use of sophisticated diagnostic instruments, pharmacology, and surgery. On the Indian view, however, healing involves transformations not only of matter but also of spirit, and healing incorporates self-knowledge and self-transformation, guided by essential elements of Indian value, such as cultivation of one's inherent awareness, and the uncovering of one's ultimate Self-nature.

> . . . yoga and other practices are helping to change our whole concept of health and restoring the broken link between medicine and spirituality. As the modern practitioner finds himself more and more helpless in the face of purely functional disorders, we seem to be on the eve of a medical revolution, which should restore the lost balance and do way, among other things, with excessive reliance on drugs.[9]

Classical Yoga is a source of many specific concepts and practices that promote well-being, psychophysical and spiritual. Further, Yoga is a paradigmatic system of religious therapeutics—a path of healing that serves the purpose of religious liberation. Among world traditions, classical Yoga is a useful starting point for inquiry into the relationship of medical and religious health because it connects the cultivation of physical and psychological health with spiritual well-being and exemplifies the idea of religious liberation as healing.

In the Indian religious and philosophical traditions in general, the human body is considered different from the true Self that is eligible for liberation. Body and mind are generally considered as a unity, and an ontological distinction is drawn between body/mind and Self, rather than between body and mind, as Western traditions tend to do.[10] Consonant with the Indian view, I use the term *psychophysical* to refer to states and processes of embodied human life. This term distinguishes the domain of body/mind from that of the ultimate Self. Indian philosophy is often stereotyped as strictly dualistic as regards body and Self. In particular,

Sāṃkhya and classical Yoga have dualistic ontologies, with consciousness and materiality as the two primordial forms of being. However, investigation of the relation of spirituality and healing in Yoga and other Indian traditions reveals a range of interpretations of the relation of body and Self. As regards concepts of health, Western thinking tends to regard health in physical and psychological terms, but Indian views of person and body substantiate a broader interpretation of health, embracing religious and other dimensions of well-being, and demonstrating a closer relation between medical and religious concerns.

Psychophysical health is integral to Yoga's religious path, but even more important is the healing that constitutes liberation: the prevailing of a person's true nature, and the overcoming of limitations and suffering. Classical Yoga is a system of self-cultivation enjoined for the attainment of liberation, and progress on Yoga's religious path is a process of healing (recovering the wholeness) of one's true nature. Liberation as actualization of unobstructed self-identity, and, consequently, the elimination of suffering, constitute achievement of the health of the person in her or his fundamental nature. While cultivation of body and health is not an end, but a means in classical Yoga, Yoga makes a significant contribution to our understanding of health and the relationship of health and religiousness. This study offers a model of religious therapeutics, based on analysis of body and health in Āyurveda, classical Yoga, and Tantra. Relations between healing and spiritual life are treated within the two following broad categories:

1. Health in its ordinary meaning, pertaining to physical and psychological well-being.
2. Liberation as healing in an ultimate sense.

A MODEL OF RELIGIOUS THERAPEUTICS

Religious therapeutics in classical Yoga operate from a concept of the person as having a psychophysical and a spiritual dimension. Each of these dimensions is subject to healing; in short, to overcoming problems that restrict well-being and vitality, produce suffering, and interfere with the prevailing of the person's true nature. Both psychophysical and spiritual meanings of health are instrumental in classical Yoga. As regards *psychophysical health*, this study focuses on the soteriological role of body and health in Yoga and argues that the refined awareness, discipline, and cultivation of the body/mind are integral to Yogic religious life, and prepare one for the higher stages of cultivation of consciousness leading to liberation. Presentation of classical Yoga as a paradigm of religious therapeutics addresses both somatic and spiritual experience, focusing on these two main themes:

1. Although body and psychophysical health are of instrumental and not ultimate value in classical Yoga, body and health have significant soteriological functions.
2. Liberation in Yoga is healing in an ultimate sense. It concerns attainment of well-being with respect to the human being's most fundamental nature and highest soteriological potential.

Because the word 'health' is ordinarily used to denote physical, psychological or psychophysical well-being, it might seem that the use of 'health' in reference to spiritual well-being is a metaphorical application of the term. However, there are grounds for broadening the extension of the term 'health' to apply to the well-being and freedom from suffering of the whole person. If the human being is considered to be more than a psychophysical entity (as is the case in Yoga, where *puruṣa* or consciousness is held to be the person's true nature), then it is legitimate to speak of health with respect to this spiritual Self, and of ultimate liberation from suffering as healing. Self-identity is a significant determinant of both psychophysical and spiritual well-being. This idea is suggested by Wilhelm Halbfass, who identifies the recovery of self-identity and well-being as a point of connection between psychophysical healing and religious liberation.[11] The concept of *liberation as healing* utilizes meanings of health revealed by analysis of Āyurvedic determinants of health, and explores metaphysical conceptions of personhood—such as freedom and identity—in their medical and soteriological implications. A model of religious therapeutics is presented below with eight branches. The first five areas, based on classical Yoga's eight limbs, provide an initial matrix of religious therapeutics. A more comprehensive model is established by incorporating the traditions of Āyurveda and Tantra. The Āyurvedic view of the person differs significantly from classical Yoga's position that body and Self are utterly distinct. Āyurveda adds the dimension of *medical therapeutics* within a holistic context of embodied and spiritual life. In Tantra, body can be understood as a vehicle to enlightenment, and as enlightenable itself. Tantra adds to an evolving model of religious therapeutics the dimension of *aesthetics*, incorporating sacred and healing music,

Branches of Religious Therapeutics

1. Metaphysical and epistemic foundations
2. Soteriology (theory of salvation or liberation)
3. Value theory and ethics
4. Physical practice
5. Cultivation of consciousness
6. Medicine and health-care
7. Aesthetics
8. Community

dance, and art. Unlike classical Yoga, Tantra esteems nature, human physicality, the feminine, and relationality. Classical Yoga, Tantra, and Āyurveda are featured here in part because their somatic orientations make their therapeutic dimensions more palpable. These three traditions are in many ways iconoclastic within the larger context of Hindu views of the body, and therefore they are especially interesting for extending our insight into body and religiousness. Finally, Āyurveda, Tantra, and other world traditions expand the model of religious therapeutics with the notion of *community:* relationality and communication in the domains of nature, culture, and the sacred.

Chapter 1, "Body and Philosophies of Healing," examines Anglo-European and Indian assumptions, setting the stage for analysis of the meaning of health, and supporting the claim that 'health' is properly predicated of the *person*, not the body or body/mind only. Chapter 2, "Meanings of Health in Āyurveda," presents determinants of health derived from the text *Caraka-saṃhitā,* and its commentary *Āyurveda-dīpikā*. Āyurveda has a comprehensive view of health as a positive state. It is concerned with physical more than spiritual well-being, yet it is grounded in Hindu religio-philosophical principles, and expands the model of religious therapeutics by providing a system of health-maintenance and medicine within a religious context. Fifteen determinants of health are discussed under four headings: (1) biological and ecological, (2) medical and psychological, (3) sociocultural and aesthetic, and (4) metaphysical and religious. Criticism may be lodged against the Indian emphasis on spirituality to the extent that mundane well-being is neglected, but Āyurveda is an antidote to such a criticism, with its focus on healthful life as holy life.

Chapter 3, "Classical Yoga as a Religious Therapeutic," analyzes Patañjali's *Yoga-sūtras* and its commentaries *Yoga-bhāṣya* and *Tattva-viśāradī* to present a matrix of classical Yoga as a system of religious therapeutics. This analysis shows Yoga's stance on meanings of health in the psychophysical and the spiritual dimensions of human life, and explores connections between Yoga's therapeutic and soteriological elements. Determinants of health excavated from Āyurveda illuminate the ultimate soteriological healing that Yoga offers: the concepts of wholeness, identity, and freedom integral to psychophysical health are operative in metaphysical and soteriological domains as well. Classical Yoga's most significant feature as a religious therapeutic is that liberation is healing: the curing of limitations and suffering in an ultimate sense.

Chapter 4, "Tantra and Aesthetic Therapeutics," draws on the tradition of Tantra, particularly the texts *Mahānirvāṇa Tantra* and *Ṣaṭ-cakra-nirūpāṇa* to add *aesthetics* as a dimension of religious therapeutics. As an example of comparative inquiry into religious therapeutics, I discuss sacred music as a religious therapeutic in several Asian and Native American traditions. In the conclusion, "Community: Relationality in Religious Therapeutics," the model of religious therapeutics is supplemented with the dimension of *community*, incorporating ecological, social, and religious relationality and communication.

Inquiry into religious therapeutics can address particular traditions, or be done comparatively. One line of inquiry is investigation of particular themes such as sacred music, or meditation practices, or ways of praying for healing. Another approach is examination of entire traditions or sects, in order to excavate their therapeutic concerns and contributions. Inquiry into medicine and religion in world traditions benefits from collaborative effort. Here I offer initial steps toward identifying relations among body, health, and religiousness, finding the Indian tradition fertile ground for accomplishing the main purpose of this study: establishing foundations of an interpretive model of religious therapeutics.

Chapter One

Body and Philosophies of Healing

Investigation of health and religiousness requires inquiry into ways of understanding the body. Human beings are embodied beings, and must come to terms with their physicality in the process of realizing their spiritual potential. This chapter examines concepts of body, showing how they ground philosophies of healing, with Anglo-European approaches providing a comparative context for Hindu views. Hindu concepts of the body are represented here by classical Yoga, Tantra, and Āyurveda, systems that are unusual in the Hindu tradition because of the priority they give, in different ways, to the body. The spiritually oriented healing paths offered by these three traditions together provide a model of religious therapeutics, useful for interpreting relations between healing and spirituality in world traditions.

BODY IN WESTERN PHILOSOPHY OF MEDICINE

Presuppositions about the Body

Among the root philosophical presuppositions of the Anglo-European tradition is Plato's concept of the person, from which arises his exhortation to purify the soul (by means of a philosophical therapeutic) from the prison-house of the body. The body, according to Plato, is the source of obstacles to attainment of pure, rational consciousness—obstacles such as maintenance demands, sensual distraction, sickness and pain, and motivation toward conflict and war.[1] Nietzsche speaks from the modern period to recognize one of the great mistakes of the Western philosophical tradition: "They despised the body: they left it out of the account: more, they treated it as an enemy."[2] Nietzsche inverts Platonic idealism, and against "the despisers of the body" voices a counter-exhortation to recognize the body's wisdom:

> Behind your thoughts and feelings, my brother, stands a mighty commander, an unknown sage—he is called Self. He lives in your body, he is your body.[3]

Nietzsche calls for a redress of the Western philosophical orientation operative since Plato, in which body is opposed to mind, mind is valorized, and body is overlooked or maligned. Significant among Western concepts of the body are Plato's prison-house, the New Testament characterization of the body as a temple, and the seventeenth-century scientific view of body as machine, epitomized in the thought of Descartes. In these notions of the human body, the metaphor of body as *container* is dominant. Plato initiated the tradition with the prison-house metaphor, and Christianity contributed the influential image of the body as a temple:

> What? Know ye not that your body is the temple of the Holy Ghost which is in you, which ye have of God, and ye are not your own? For ye are bought with a price, therefore glorify God in your body, and in your spirit, which are God's.
>
> 1 Corinthians 6:19–20

This New Testament passage presents a dichotomous concept of person as composed of spirit contained in body, which implies both the sacredness of body, and its subsidiary position as a vessel for the spirit. Eliot Deutsch points out that the temple metaphor is prescriptive, telling us how we *ought* to regard our bodies: "It finds its intelligibility within a religious framework of values that sees the possibility of a reverential attitude toward all things in virtue of their divine origin and grounding."[4] Indeed, this message from First Corinthians is a cornerstone of codes of health-ethics in many Christian denominations, including, for instance, the prohibiting of tobacco use. The metaphor of the body as the temple of the Holy Spirit grounds an important element of Christian religious therapeutics: The body is not only given by God, but it serves as the abode of the Holy Spirit, instantiated as the individual's spirit. Thus to neglect the body or to engage in activities damaging to it would be sacrilege.

'Container' images of the body are consistent with the speculated etymological association of the English term 'body' with the Old High German *botahha:* 'tub,' 'vat' or 'cask.'[5] Classical Chinese thought offers a concept of the body entirely different from the 'container' image. Roger

T. Ames writes that in classical Chinese thought, "mind and body are polar rather than dualistic concepts, and as such, can only be understood in relation to each other," and that "'person' is properly regarded as a 'psychosomatic process.'"[6] 'Polarism' is a symbiotic relation, a unity of two mutually dependent processes that require one another in order for each to be what it is. Dualism, on the other hand, implies the coexistence of two factors of fundamentally different natures, such as Plato's *psyche* and *soma*, Descartes' thinking substance and extended substance, or Yoga's *prakṛti* (consciousness) and *puruṣa* (materiality). Underlying classical Chinese polarism is the presupposition of a single order of being, wherein various objects and processes differ not in kind, but in degree. Related to Chinese polarism is a commitment to process ontology rather than substance ontology, producing an organismic interpretation of the world as composed of interdependent and intrinsically related processes. The combination of Chinese process metaphysics with a polar conception of the psychic and the somatic yields a holistic notion of 'person' as a *psychosomatic process*. An important implication of this concept of person is its circumvention of the main problem faced by dualistic accounts of the person, the problem of how two fundamentally different substances—such as consciousness and matter—can interact.

Deutsch observes that the dominant Western metaphors of body, besides being 'container' images, are generally dualistic and conceptually static. That is, it is assumed that the body is an objective given of nature or experience, and that the meaning of 'body' can be spelled out in purely descriptive terms. Deutsch argues that the meanings of 'personhood' and 'body' are found not in descriptive terms, but in terms of *achievement*. Person and body can be understood not just as givens of nature, but in terms of self-cultivation—how an individual appropriates and integrates the conditions of his or her being:

> *My* body *is* only as it is articulated within my being as a person. The isolable physical conditions of my individual being, in other words, are not my body. What I recognize as integral to me qua person is not this configuration but what, in a way, I have made of it as my own.[7]

An interpretation of person and body as *achievement concepts* is an antidote to 'container' concepts of the body, and grounds an understanding of the person in which body is integral. The metaphysics of René Descartes (1596–1650) is paradigmatic of the Anglo-European view of rationality as central to personhood, and mind as separate from and superior to body.

Descartes on Body and Medicine

Descartes' dualistic metaphysics postulates two fundamental substances, thinking substance and extended substance, and thus he relegates the human being to a schizoid state, where the mind is valorized and the body is considered a material object, analyzable in terms of mechanistic science. The Cartesian legacy, in the words of Maxine Sheets-Johnstone, "has been not only to divide the fundamental integrity of creaturely life, but to depreciate the role of the living body in knowing and making sense of the world, in learning, in the creative arts, and in self- and interpersonal understandings."[8] As we enter the twenty-first century, the redress of philosophical and functional implications of Descartes' casting of the 'mind-body problem' incorporates phenomenological and non-Western approaches to our understanding of person and body. This redress incorporates a range of disciplines including philosophy, anthropology, and linguistics, and generates criticism in medical and social theory.

The damaging social effects of Cartesianism supply compelling reasons to challenge it: "This hierarchical dualism has been used to subserve projects of oppression directed toward women, animals, nature, and other 'Others.'"[9] *The Absent Body*, by physician and philosopher Drew Leder, offers a phenomenological account of how Cartesian-type dualism, while misguided and misguiding, is experientially persuasive, owing to our usual state of forgetfulness of our embodiment. Descartes, whose thought was conditioned by, and contributed to, a mechanistic view of person and world, was extremely interested in the philosophy of medicine. Descartes names the philosophy of medicine as his foremost concern in his first published work, *Discourse on Method* (1637):

> . . . I have resolved to devote the rest of my life to nothing other than trying to acquire some knowledge of nature from which we may derive rules in medicine which are more reliable than those we have had up till now. Moreover, my inclination makes me so strongly opposed to all other projects, and especially those which can be useful to some persons only by harming others, that if circumstances forced me to engage in any such pursuit, I do not think I would be capable of succeeding in it.[10]

Another of Descartes' statements pertinent to his interest in medical philosophy is found in his letter to William Cavendish (1645): "The preservation of health has always been the principle end of my studies."[11] Descartes considered his medical philosophy as an application of his physics, which grounds both his medical philosophy and his ethical theory. According to Richard B. Carter, Descartes "envisioned a social revolution based on his philosophy of medicine."[12] Descartes endeavored to apply his science of nature to human beings as objects accessible by the same principles as physical objects. With consideration of how humans use institutions for self-preservation, he claimed that his science of nature could explain the constitution of a "body politic" as ethical to the extent that it accords with the natural principles of cosmogenesis and embryogenesis.[13] Descartes was concerned to demonstrate that the self is a thinking being, devoid of spatial characteristics, and is capable of existing independently of the body. The entire title of Descartes' *Meditations* is *Meditations on First Philosophy, in which are demonstrated the existence of God and the distinction between the human soul and body*. None of the *Mediations*, however, treats the living body in detail, though the human body is a predominant theme in other works of Descartes, notably his *Discourse on Method* (1637) (published posthumously in 1664), and his final work, *Passions of the Soul* (1649). The second meditation is entitled "The nature of the human mind and that it is more easily known than the body." This meditation does not in fact discuss the nature of the *human* body, but rather addresses the nature of *physical* bodies and our knowledge of them. By way of example, Descartes presents the case of a piece of beeswax, which, after melting, loses its particular shape, color, scent, and resonance, and retains only its extension in space. Spatial extension is known by reason, not by the senses. Descartes regarded extension as the essential property of objects in the category of substance he calls matter, *res extensa* (extended stuff), and distinct from the category of substance he calls mind, *res cogitans* (thinking stuff).

Descartes' physics is concerned with 'body' in general, that is, *substance,* of which particular physical 'bodies' are composed. His physical theory of the generation of the cosmos provided paradigms for both his medical theory of the embryogenesis of the human body and his ethical theory of the generation of a healthy "body politic." His medical philosophy applies principles of his mathematical physics of general body to the living human body, each of which is united with a soul. Descartes conceived the anatomy of the human body from the standpoint of its fitness to carry out the intellectual operations of the mind. In the same way that medicine is the science of maintaining the human body's organization so that it can carry out the operations of the mind, ethics, in Descartes' view, is the science of maintaining the organized cooperation of groups of persons as a political body.[14] In the opening paragraph of his *Description of the Human Body,* Descartes expresses the view that both ethics and medicine are informed by our knowledge of ourselves, specifically of the respective functions of soul and body.[15] Descartes' letters to his Jesuit disciple Père Mesland distinguish physical body from human body on the basis of the human body's "disposition" to receive the human soul. The first letter (1645) stipulates that body in general means "a determined part of matter, and at the same time, the quantity of matter of which the universe in composed." Descartes next states that what is meant by "human body" is not a determinate portion of matter, but "all the matter that is united together with the soul of man . . . and we believe that this body is whole while it has all the dispositions required for conserving this union."[16] In the *Meditations,* Descartes supports his view that the self is incorporeal by applying methodological doubt. In doubting everything that can be doubted in order to seek an indubitable starting point for knowledge, Descartes surmises that anything spatial could be produced by a dream, or by the deceptive work of an evil genius. He concludes that he himself must exist in order to be doubting in the first place, and, from there, he argues that "since he must exist despite the supposition that everything corporeal or spatial is but a dream or a demonic hoax, he cannot himself be anything spatial or corporeal."[17]

Princess Elizabeth of Bohemia challenged Descartes in a letter with a question about how the soul, a thinking substance, can interact with the body when they have nothing in common (20 June 1643). Descartes' reply about an "inexplicable union between body and soul" is unsatisfactory to her, and in a subsequent letter (13 September 1645), she requests that Descartes give "a definition of the passions."[18] Albert A. Johnstone notes that Elizabeth questions Descartes about the influence of emotional turmoil on clear philosophical thinking, and suggests that her criticisms "point toward the necessity of introducing feeling, and hence the body, into the concept of the self."[19] Body for Descartes is the seen body, not the felt body. In ruminating on his experimentally derived conclusion that he must exist as a thing that thinks, Descartes asks, "What is this 'I' that necessarily exists?"

> Well, the first thought to come to mind was that I had a face, hands, arms, and the whole mechanical structure of limbs which can be seen in a corpse, and which I called the body.[20]

Descartes conceives body in terms of its appearance, not from the standpoint of what later philosophers have called 'the subjective body,' 'the felt body,' or 'the tactile-kinesthetic body.' Merleau-Ponty contributed to the phenomenology of the experienced body, distinguishing between the objective 'seen' body and the subjective 'experienced body.'

> . . . we must learn to distinguish it [the experienced body] from the objective body as set forth in works on physiology. This is not the body, which is capable of being inhabited by a consciousness. . . . It is simply a question of recognizing that the body, as a chemical structure of an agglomeration of tissues, is formed by a process of reduction, from the primordial phenomenon of the body-for-us, the body of experience, or the perceived body.[21]

Tracing the evolution of the concept of the body through the history of Western medicine shows that Descartes' 'mechanical body' dominates early modern medical thinking, and that the 'experienced body' emerges as significant in contemporary medical philosophy.

Body in the History of Western Medicine

The history of medicine is a conceptual history of the body. Approaches to understanding and treating the sick body become culturally engrained habits of thought, which in turn engender a metaphysical *Zeitgeist* or 'Spirit of the Age,' claims Sheets-Johnstone. Western medical theory for the 2000 years prior to the Enlightenment and scientific revolution was based on the Greek humoral theory articulated by Hippocrates of Cos in the fifth century B.C.E. A medieval text, *Regimen Sanitarius Salernum,* originating around 1140 C.E. from the School of Salernum, the leading European center for medical study, discusses humoral theory and provides evidence of its prevailing from the ancient period. Greek humoral theory was grounded on Empedocles' theory of the four elements: air, fire, earth, and water, and their basic qualities: cold, heat, dryness, and moistness. Onto the schema of the four elements, Hippocrates mapped the four elements of living things: blood, phlegm, yellow bile, and black bile. Thus he formulated a medical theory grounded in metaphysics wherein body and cosmos are coterminous.[22]

Ancient Greek diagnostic and therapeutic methods, like those of India's Āyurvedic medicine, address the proportionality of elements constituting both patient and medicinal and pathogenic substances. As in Āyurveda, the goal of diagnosis in the Hippocratic tradition "was to obtain a total unified picture of the patient's condition . . . because the whole body was felt to be involved in any ill that befell it."[23] In both ancient medical traditions, therapeutic restoration of the proper harmonic relationships among elements and their qualities emphasized the patient's diet, regimen, and environmental, seasonal, and interpersonal circumstances. In Greece as in India, the doctrine of humors is a medical formulation of a cosmic physiology dominated by the themes of circulation of fluids and a chain of successive 'cookings' of nutriment by the sun, the cooking fire, and the digestion. The divergence of the ancient Greco-Latin and Indian medical traditions is Āyurveda's conceptualization of a vast combinative system of humors and qualities. This system consists in enormous catalogues of medicinal substances. Greek and Latin science, by contrast, produced a natural history wherein abstraction was not *combinative* and *ampliative*, but rather *classificatory*, involving the reduction of specifications.[24] However, there is remarkable similarity between Greek and Indian views of the patient not merely as a body, but as person with a consciousness and unique circumstances, who is physically and in other ways part of the world. On such an interpretation of the person, the healing art is concerned with restoring equilibrium within the patient and between patient and environment, and potentiating the body's innate power to heal.

Classical Western medicine (that of ancient Greece, and the European Middle Ages and Renaissance) regarded the body as "an abstract nomenclatural construct . . . a subtle body of humours and dispositions; but the perception of its 'nature' conformed more to a classificatory aesthetic than to the truth of its observable condition."[25] In the early modern period beginning in the seventeenth century, the rise of empirical science meant a revolutionary change in medicine's approach to the body, symbolized by the study of cadavers, and marked by an emphasis on the concrete structure of the body regarded as an intricately complex machine. While ancient Western medicine held the body to be a sacred entity—and like ancient Chinese and Indian thought—considered the human body a microcosm corresponding to the whole cosmological order, the early modern scientific approach relegated the body to the status of profane flesh to be empirically analyzed. While ancient etiological theory thought in terms of the balance and imbalance of qualities within a pre-established system of categories, early modern medicine replaced the schemes of qualities with the principle of causal agency. A paradigmatic example of medicine's success in refining the principle of causal agency is the understanding and controlling of bacterial disease, based on Pasteur's nineteenth-century discovery of bacterial pathogenicity.

The body, illness, and health were radically reconceptualized in the Western world in the sixteenth century. With Vesalius' discoveries in anatomy and, in the seventeenth century, William Harvey's explanation of the circulation of blood within a closed loop, there was a progressive materialization of the body, as structures and functions were "*organ-ized* into discrete functional systems."[26] ('Modern' or Western scientific medicine was introduced to India during this same period, when the Portuguese conquered Goa in 1510 and established a hospital there.)[27] The mechanistic thinking of early modern medicine remains influential in contemporary medicine. The materialist conception of the body prevalent in contemporary Western medical theory is accompanied by a physicochemical orientation to the person and to therapeutics, which Sheets-Johnstone says "eventuates in both an eroded sense of self and an eroded sense of responsibility."[28] She lodges the criticism that the paradigm of localization-in-place of the various organs and systems underlies present-day Western medicine's organization according to various specializations. This organization contributes to the tendency to treat particular parts of the body without much consideration of their relations to other parts, nor to the health of the whole body and person.

Ancient Western science was holistic, and Āyurvedic and Chinese medicine have remained so from ancient times. However, while Sheets-Johnstone is correct to identify a trend of increasing "materialization" of the body in the history of medicine, her account omits postmodern discourse on the body in the context of medicine, a discourse informed by new cooperating technologies and epistemic approaches. The body as a discursive formation in Western medical history has evolved through a number of models. Levin and Solomon identify the ancient period's *rational body* based on an aesthetic of matrices of dynamic qualities. Next are analytic medicine's *anatomical, physiological,* and *biochemical bodies* originating in the scientific progress of the early modern period. In the twentieth century, the dominant models of the body are the *psychosomatic* and the *psychoneuroimmunological.* If we consider the human body not just as a biological entity, but as a *discursive formation*, as Levin and Solomon recommend, we realize that contemporary Western medical science "has begun to restore the body to the larger world-order."[29]

The factors instrumental in the current evolution of medical theory are both scientific and philosophical. The analytic medical research of the early modern period investigated the tissues of the body with the eye and then the microscope, revealing the structure of the body not just in terms of major organs and systems, but as networks of tissues. Tissues were analyzed in terms of differentiated cellular bodies, and these in turn were probed at the atomic level, and understood in terms of molecular interactions. In the early twentieth century, there emerged *psychosomatic medicine,* which advocated the unity of mind and body, and made use of biochemistry to account for particular disorders originating in a zone between the material body and the 'volitional body' or psyche. Although psychosomatic medicine advocated the unity of mind and body, "it has failed to overcome the dualism which isolated this unity from its environment—nature, society, and culture."[30] A current discursive formation of *behavioral medicine* defends an implication of psychosomatic medicine that earlier psychosomatic medicine restricted itself from fully supporting: If 'mind' and 'body' are indeed dimensions of a unity, then *all* diseases are in some respect psychosomatic, that is, they affect both body and mind. Psychosomatic medicine, however, restricted itself to a limited number of syndromes, for instance, allergy and hypertension, and to a narrow range of mediating instances, notably the tracing of particular diseases to specific personality characteristics.

Behavioral medicine, informed by knowledge of psychoneuroimmunology and psychoneuroendocrinology, provides a new paradigm of the body that works against dualistic views of mind/body, body/environment, and individual/community. As we enter the twenty-first century, research in immunocompetence reveals a new body:

> This dynamic, synergic body is seen as a system network functioning in a larger system, a multifactoral network of cause and effect, in which effects also become causes. The body cannot be represented as a "substance." It has become necessary to represent it, rather, as a system of intercommunicatively organized processes, functioning at different levels of differentiation and integration. It represents a growing body of evidence supporting a *new concept of disease* and a much broadened understanding of epidemiology, according to which diseases do not take place in an environment conditioned only by the forces of nature, but occur, rather, in a *communicative field* [italics added], a world of social, cultural, and historical influences: influences which the proprioceptive body processes as meanings.[31]

The body as conceived by psychoneuroimmunology resonates with the *Bhagavadgītā's* body as a field within a web of countless other interacting fields, and the Āyurvedic articulation of the body as *saṃyogavahin,* 'a vehicle for congruous junctions.' Contemporary medical philosophy that dissolves dualisms pertaining to personhood invokes principles consonant with those underlying India's ancient religio-philosophical systems.

There is yet another concept of body emerging in the current evolution of Western medicine, a concept informed by both scientific and philosophical discourse. This is the *body of experienced meaning,* a model of the body that permits accounts of how the processes of disease and healing are related to proprioceptively experienced meanings. The success of establishing correlations between the patient's phenomenological or experienced body, and the states of that person's medical body, depends on more than medical knowledge. It also requires patients' abilities to "fine-tune their embodied awareness, their sensitivity to processes of bodily experiencing, and their skillfulness in carrying those processes forward into more articulate, more discriminating meanings."[32]

The emerging awareness of the *experienced body* in the philosophical thinking that bears on medicine may be informed by the Indian tradition's guiding principle of cultivation of self-knowledge. Yoga, Āyurveda, and Tantra offer conceptual grounds and practical means of cultivating self-knowledge in the domain of health. The extension of the term health can be broadened from its usual application to physical and psychological well-being, to encompass freedom from limitations and from suffering of the whole person, inclusive of the human being's spiritual dimension. Concepts of person and body are fundamental to the philosophy and practice of healing arts that serve the purpose of human well-being conceived as broadly as possible. What is called for, according to Sheets-Johnstone, is neither extreme materialization of the body nor extreme animism. Similarly, medicine and the healing arts benefit from deeper consideration of both scientific and spiritual dimensions of human life.

ICONOCLASTIC CONCEPTS OF BODY IN YOGA, TANTRA, AND ĀYURVEDA

Traditional Indian Views of Person and Body

Hegel's claim that "man . . . has not been posited in India" is the point of departure for Wilhelm Halbfass' discussion of person and self *in Tradition and Reflection: Explorations in Indian Thought.* Halbfass concludes that the idea of the human being as a rational animal, and as a being capable of apprehending the future, has been articulated in Indian thought. However, owing to the soteriological orientation of Indian philosophy, this particular concept of man is not central in the way that it is in Western thought.[33]

The Sanskrit word for human being, *manuṣya,* is derived from the verbal root *man,* 'to think,' which is also the root of the noun *manas,* 'mind.' In Hindu texts, the word *manuṣya* is not as common nor as significant as the word *ātman:* the Self and immortal essence inherent in all living entities.[34] It is the *ātman* and not the human being as *homo sapiens* that is to be liberated.[35] *Ātman* is common to all living beings, yet there is another way that the human being is not-different from other beings: all are subject to *saṃsāra,* transmigratory existence through innumerable births and deaths. Transitions are possible among existences as supra-human, human, animal, and plant. But the human being has a special and perhaps exclusive soteriological qualification or *adhikāra,* the capacity for liberative knowledge. Liberative knowledge is knowledge that permits discovery or realization of one's true nature, and freedom from the cycle of *saṃsāra.* In view of this special qualification the *Mahābhārata* says that none is higher than the human being. The potential for religious liberation is a critical factor in Indian views of person, body, and self.

Sanskrit terms for the human body include *śarīram* and *dehaḥ.* Both of these words reflect the predominant Indian view that the body is not the person's true and fundamental nature. *Śarīram* is derived from the verbal root √ *ṣr,* 'to break': the body ultimately breaks apart. The word *dehaḥ* suggests an envelope; it derives from the verbal root √ *dih*, 'to cover,' alluding to the cloak or container of the immaterial Self. John M. Koller identifies, among the details of India's many subtraditions, two common features of concepts of the body:

1. Body is really body/mind, and an ontological line is drawn between body/mind and Self.
2. The body/mind is not a static entity, but a karmic process:

   . . . constituted by interaction with the other processes in an ever-widening sphere that extends ultimately to the whole world, linking each person to other persons and beings in a web of interconnections that extends to all times and places.[36]

While the Western philosophical tradition has tended to oppose mind and body, the Indian view of the person begins with the presumption of integrated psychophysiological functioning: "seeing the body as conscious and consciousness as bodily activity."[37] The body/mind complex is rejected as the real Self, and similar to the Anglo-European struggle to reconcile body and mind, the Indian traditions have the problem of relating body/mind to Self. While the Anglo-European traditions are interested in the problem primarily from a philosophical standpoint, the Indian concern for the problem is soteriological.

Two Indian traditions reject—on different grounds and with different implications—the existence of a Self beyond the lived body/mind. They are both *nāstika*, that is, not among the Veda-accepting (*āstika*) systems. In Buddhism, a non-substantialist view of the human psychophysical entity replaces a notion of 'Self.' In Cārvaka, the materialist *darśana*, the body and self are considered identical. Cārvaka (also known as Lokāyata) differs from Western materialism in that Cārvāka considers the body to be imbued with consciousness.[38]

Ancient Indian interpretations of the person do not entirely exclude simple mind-body dualism. The *Maitri Upaniṣad* refers to the tranquil eternal one by whom "this body is set up in intelligence . . . (and) who propels it" (Mait. Up. 2.3–4). The *Bṛhadāraṇyaka Upaniṣad* says the "knowing self" or "breathing self" has entered the bodily self (*śarīra ātman)* as fire is put into a fire receptacle (Bṛhad. Up. 1.4.7).[39] The *nāstika* tradition of Jainism holds a more radically dualistic account of the person than these Upaniṣadic conceptions: The soul, *jīva,* pervades the body and is spatially coextensive with it, because the soul's indefinitely many space points (*pradeśa*) precisely assume the dimensions of the corporeal form they occupy.[40]

Body in the Vedas

Vedic conceptions of the human nature were embedded in mythic and ritualistic contexts. The climate of the *Vedas* is more earthly and temporal than that of Upaniṣadic and subsequent Indian thought, and in the *Vedas*, humans are treated more as earthly, temporal beings. In Vedic usage, the words *ātman* and *puruṣa* tend to refer to the embodied person, rather than to the absolute spiritual Self. A frequently used Vedic term for person is *jīvā*. Etymolgically, *ātman* means 'breath' and *jīva* means 'life.' Troy Wilson Organ identifies a variety of usages of *ātman* and *jīva*. The word *jīva* is used in the *Ṛgveda* to designate living, breathing beings, for example, "Rise, woman and go to the world of living beings (*jīvas*)" [RV 10:2.2.8]. The term *ātman* is pivotal in a Ṛgvedic cremation prayer to Agni that indicates belief in a Self different from the body: "Agni, consume him not entirely. . . . Let the eye repair to the sun, the breath (*ātman*) to the wind" [RV 10:1.16.3]. Besides denoting breath, *ātman* can denote the body, as in these healing hymns:

> The virtues of the plants which are desirous of bestowing wealth issue from them, man, towards thy body (*ātman*) like cattle from a pen.
>
> RV 10:8.7.8

> I banish disease from each limb, from each hair, from each joint where it is generated, from thy whole person (*ātman*).
>
> RV 10:12.12.5–6

Ātman also denotes life as existence in the *Ṛgveda*, for example, in thanks given to Indra for bestowing existence on human beings [RV 1:1.11.8]. *Ātman* also implies the vitality of the life-force: "May he, the bull, be the impregnator of the perpetual plants, for in him is the *ātman* of the fixed and the movable worlds" [RV 7:6.12.6]. Often the word *ātman* is used in the *Ṛgveda* to designate essential identity: "Thou flowest, Indu (denoting Soma), the inviolable, the most exhilarating; thou art thyself (*ātman*) the best support of Indra" [RV 9:4.18.3]. An example of the term *ātman* expressing the meaning of *essential identity* (identity of something, not necessarily a person) is this passage concerning medicinal plants: "As soon as I take these plants in my hand making the sick man strong, the *ātman* of the malady perishes" [RV 10.8.7.11].

Vedic texts, particularly the *Brāhmaṇas*, classify the human being as a *paśu*, an animal, as the preeminent animal, the ruler of all the other animals, and the only animal able to perform ritual and sacrifice. The human being is *sukṛta*, 'well-made,' and, according to the *Atharvaveda*, is distinguished by having ritual powers, access to sacred texts, and power to influence the universe. These powers come from the human being's unique association with *Brahman*, the supreme principle [AV 10:2]. However, the Vedic classification of the human being as a member of the animal kingdom, based largely on physical similarity, demonstrates a body-oriented view of the person. Further evidence of a body-oriented view of the person is present in the Vedic perspective on the human being as agent of ritual and sacrificial acts. Yet a pervasive theme in Vedic views of person is religious holism: body and consciousness are both instruments of agency, particularly sacrificial agency. In the vision of the Vedic *ṛṣis* or seers, no dualism exists in their understanding of person: consciousness has body as its locus, and the body's volitional actions are entirely dependent on the consciousness.[41]

The human being's superior intelligence, discernment, and expression are noted in the *Aitareya Āraṇyaka*. A significant application of the human power to know, and our distinctness from other animals, is our consciousness of the future. The ability to 'know the tomorrow' (*veda śvasthanam*) is a necessary component of man's soteriological prerogative. *Mokṣa*, freedom from worldly limitations, is achieved by ritual action informed by knowledge of *dharma*. Acting according to *dharma* (righteousness) requires comprehension of the temporal horizons within which *dharma* has meaning. In Vedic thought, man's capacity to understand *dharma* grounds human beings' soteriological mandate and opportunity. The human being as rational animal has powers superior to those of other animals, but in the Hindu context, man's highest potential is not the exercise of this power in dominion of the earth and its creatures. In fact, such dominion is undesirable. Man's privilege is to become liberated from the world, not master of it. Our mandate is not to make use of other beings, but to use our own human existence as a vehicle of transcendence.[42] The theme of self-transcendence evolves with various paths of self-cultivation—yogic and otherwise—for the purpose of liberation.

Body in the Upaniṣads

The *Upaniṣads* contain a range of understandings of the body, most of them within organic, holistic accounts of the person, showing the person's fundamental nature, *ātman*, to be non-different from the one Absolute, *Brahman*. An illustration is the instruction of Śvetaketu by his father, who imparts that the One, having longed to become many, diversified into the elements fire, water, and earth, and entered these elements as *ātman*. *Ātman* is the ground of all manifest things, just as clay is the basis of various clay objects [Chānd. Up. Bk. 6]. A view of the self as having both an individual and a universal aspect is expressed in the allegory of the two birds in a tree, one eating fruit, the other abstaining and looking on [Muṇḍ. Up. 3:3.1.1; Śvet. Up. 4]. The bird who eats is the individual embodied self, given to enjoyment and suffering, the other is the true Self, the universal and knowing *Brahman*.

In the *Taittirīya Upaniṣad*, the very body of Brahman is the source of creation of human beings:

> From this Self (*Brahman*) space arose; from space, wind; from wind, fire; from fire, water; from water, the earth; from the earth, herbs; from herbs, food; from food, semen and ova, and from semen and ova, the person (*puruṣa*).
>
> Tait. Up. 2.1

Next, the *upaniṣad* presents the widely employed *pañca-kośa* or five-sheaths model of the person, whose core and source is *ātman*. The five sheaths (*pañca*, 'five'; *kośa,* 'sheath') are conceived as enveloping one another, and at their center is the true Self. The outermost sheath is the *body of food,* or the material body, which is filled successively with the sheath or body of *prāṇā*, *breath* (life-force), then *mind*, *consciousness*, and, at the center, *bliss*. The sheath of bliss is interpreted as either identical to, or containing, the innermost true Self, the *ātman*. The upaniṣadic five-sheath doctrine is accepted by Vedānta and many post-classical schools of Yoga, but not by classical Yoga itself. An image of the body more consonant with that of classical Yoga is given in the *Maitri Upaniṣad*.

> Sir, in this ill-smelling, unsubstantial body, which is a conglomerate of bone, skin, muscle, marrow, flesh, semen, blood, mucus, tears, rheum, feces, urine, wind, bile, and phlegm, what is the good of enjoyment of desires? In this body, which is afflicted with desire, anger, covetousness, delusion, fear, despondency, envy, separation from the desirable, union with the undesirable, hunger, thirst, senility, death, disease, sorrow and the like, what is the good of enjoyment of desires?
>
> Mait. Up. 1:3

The *Maitri* is one of the Upaniṣads that inclines more toward dualism, thus grounding classical Sāṃkhya and Yoga, in contrast to the non-dualistic *Upaniṣads* eventuating in Vedānta. *The Maitri Upaniṣad* also incorporates elements of esoteric psychology, later incorporated in Tantra and Tāntric Yogas:

> Now, it has been said: There is a channel called the *Suṣumnā*, leading upward, conveying the breath, piercing through the palate. Through it, by joining [√*yuj*, 'to join] the breath, the syllable *Om*, and the mind, one may go aloft . . . by binding together [*saṃyoga*] the senses . . . one goes to selflessness . . . becomes a non-experiencer of pleasure and pain, he obtains the absolute unity.
>
> Mait. Up. 6.21

The *Kaṭha Upaniṣad's* enumeration of the aspects of the person is similar to that of classical Sāṃkhya and Yoga: There is nothing higher than *puruṣa*. At successively lower levels are the Unmanifest (*avyākta*), the Great Self (*Ātman*), the discriminative intellect (*buddhi*), the mind (*manas*), the senses, and the objects of sense [Kaṭh. Up. 3.10]. In addition to germs of classical Sāṃkhya and Yoga, the *Kaṭha* also contains elements of the esoteric physiology adopted and elaborated by Tantra. In a concluding verse, reference is made to the 101 *nadīs* or channels that carry *prāṇa* or life-energy, and the one that "passes up to the crown of the head"—the *Suṣumṇā* [Kaṭh. Up. 6.16].

Body in the Bhagavadgītā

The battlefield, the setting for the warrior Arjuna's instruction by Lord Kṛṣṇa, grounds the *Gītā* in a concrete world where Arjuna is at first overwhelmed by the implications of a situation in which body predominates: the physical action Arjuna chooses shall determine the physical survival or annihilation of his kinsmen in the opposing army. This dilemma occasions Kṛṣṇa's teaching that the true Self is not the body. The true Self is eternal, neither dies nor is born, but is reborn in new bodies [BhG 2.20–22].

A rich conception of the person is the *Gītā's* depiction of the body as a 'field,' and the one who knows this, "the knower of the field" [BhG 13. 1–3]. Koller describes this image as:

> . . . a field of interacting energies of different kinds and intensities, a field which is simultaneously interacting with innumerable other fields. The body-mind is a juncture or constellation of these interactions, born and reborn out of successively interacting energy-fields.[43]

Vedānta's Model of 'The Three Bodies'

Vedānta provides an important account of the person in Śaṅkara's presentation of the three bodies in the *Viveka-cūḍamaṇi*, "The Crest-Jewel of Discrimination" (eighth century C.E.). This doctrine of the three bodies is alluded to in the *Maitri Upaniṣad* [Mait. Up. 6:10]. Wimal Dissanayake gives the following explanation of the three bodies. The *gross body* (*sthūla śarīra*) is the physical body that we erroneously think is the Self. This misidentification results in part from our preoccupation with experiences of pleasure and pain as a result of contact with gross objects. The *subtle body* (*sūkṣma śarīra*), mentioned in *Maitri Upaniṣad* 6:10, can be understood in terms of dream consciousness. The contents of dream consciousness are subtle elements (*tanmātras*), which lack material properties, yet are able to influence personality and waking consciousness. The gross body is unable to understand the subtle forces of the *tanmātras*, but the subtle body can, because it is of the same nature. Thus the subtle body is responsible for the phenomenon of being at once a participant in, and a witness to, one's dream experience. *The causal or karmic body* (*kāraṇa śarīra*) is the most complex of the three bodies. It contain the *saṃskāras* or impressions of experience, which result from one's past actions. The principle of *karma* holds that all actions arise according to past conduct, and that all actions have effects in both the life of the person who acts, and in the world. Therefore, the causal body contains the possibilities of how a person's particular life experiences will manifest.[44]

Yoga's Use of the Body to Transcend Itself

In Patañjali's classical Yoga, the body is the ground of action that can lead to or obstruct liberation. Religious therapeutics in classical Yoga operate from a concept of the person as having a psychophysical and a spiritual dimension. Each of these dimensions is subject to healing; in short, to overcoming problems that restrict well-being and vitality, produce suffering, and interfere with the prevailing of the person's true nature. In classical

Yoga, the soteriological aim is realized in the freeing of *puruṣa*, consciousness, from *prakṛti*, material nature. However, among the *darśanas* or systems of Indian philosophy, Yoga is noteworthy for the integral role it accords to the body in the striving for liberation. Given Yoga's premises that (1) body and Self are entirely distinct, and (2) the soteriological goal entails the Self's independence from physicality, what can be gained by investigating Yoga's understanding of the body? The central problem of Hindu soteriology may be expressed in these two corollaries:

1. Liberation from ignorance and the suffering it produces.
2. Attainment of one's highest soteriological potential, generally conceived as realization of one's true spiritual identity.

Since human life has an inevitable physical dimension, a major challenge in seeking a spiritual goal is reconciling the physical with the spiritual, or transcending one's embodied situation to one's ultimate situation. Practice of classical or *aṣṭāṅga* (eight-fold) Yoga incorporates cultivation of the body to achieve the transcendence of embodiment. According to the *Sāṃkhya-kārikā*, which provides much of Yoga's metaphysical foundation, all things (and thus human bodies) are instantiations of the whole of creation, and may function as vehicles for attainment of the highest spiritual goal:

> From *Brahman* down to the blade of grass, the creation (*sṛṣti*) is for the benefit of the soul, until supreme knowledge is attained.
>
> SK 3.47

The *Yoga-sūtras* explain why the true Self, *puruṣa*, is associated with the human body:

> The purpose of the conjunction (*saṃyoga*) of the master [the Seer or experiencer: *puruṣa*] and the experienceable world [*prakṛti*], is the experiencer's recognition of the Self-natures of the two powers.
>
> YS 2.23

Classical Yoga understands mind and body as aspects of the psychophysical person. According to Yoga's metaphysical foundations, body, mind, and senses are all evolutes of matter, *prakṛti*. Mind/body dualism is thus avoided in Yoga, but there remains a dualism separating mind/body from consciousness. The position that 'mind' and 'body' are dimensions of a unity, rather than separate entities, grounds a pragmatically valuable orientation to etiology (the theory of disease-causation) and to treatment, by recognizing the mutual influence of physical and mental factors in health and illness. Apart from the metaphysical problems inherent in Yoga's dualism, Yoga's distinguishing mind/body from consciousness also yields an important understanding of the relation of health and religiousness: Similar to the way that mental factors have physiological consequences, and physical factors have mental consequences for health, Yoga shows that the wellness of the mind/body can assist the attainment of spiritual well-being. Conversely, the recovery of spiritual Self-nature and well-being helps to heal and vitalize the body/mind.

Because Yoga practices have health benefits, there is a misconception, particularly in the West, that health is Yoga's goal. Indian views of Yoga on the other hand, in recognizing Yoga as a religious system emphasizing the cultivation of Self-nature as consciousness, sometimes minimize the importance of body and health in Yoga. In chapter 3, I locate the soteriological role of human physicality within the context of Yoga's ultimate aim: attainment of liberation from the nature and constraints of *prakṛti*, and transcendence of the ignorance and suffering that attend material existence. Both psychophysical and spiritual meanings of health are instrumental in classical Yoga. As regards psychophysical health, the refined awareness, discipline, and cultivation of the body/mind are integral to yogic religious life, and prepare one for the higher stages of cultivation of consciousness leading to liberation. Chapter 3 presents classical Yoga as a paradigm of religious therapeutics, addressing both somatic and spiritual experience, and revealing two main principles:

1. Although body and psychophysical health are of instrumental and not ultimate value in classical Yoga, body and health have significant soteriological functions.
2. Liberation in Yoga is healing in an ultimate sense. It concerns attainment of well-being with respect to the human being's most fundamental nature and highest soteriological potential.

Tantra's Enlightenable Body

The Vedic tradition and the Tāntric tradition are distinct but interrelated currents of Indian religious culture, and they share as well as diverge in their constitutions of religious meaning. A major feature of Tantra is its ontological presupposition that the universe, and everything in it, is a manifestation of the one Brahman. Emergent from this principle is a positive attitude toward material nature and the body. The feminine principle is esteemed as the manifestation of the masculine absolute's immanent and dynamic aspect. Tantra emphasizes religious practice over theoretical knowledge, and seeks liberation through mystical knowledge gained in experience. A prominent feature of Tāntric practice is the utilization of material nature in order to transcend subjugation to materiality. Tantra regards the body as an instrument to liberation, but, more than this, considers the body as part of the sacred creation, and as capable of enlightenment. The word 'tantra' literally means 'loom' or 'that which is woven.' Its verbal root is √ *tan*, 'to stretch,' 'to expand.' Thus it carries the meaning of *expansion*—of being, of knowing, of bliss. Tantra's connotation of *expansion* recalls Wilfred Cantwell Smith's thought about the sacred as something 'more.' Diane B. Obenchain explains:

> . . . religion might be defined generally as giving care to, paying heed to, paying attention to, more *in* human life than meets the eye. What is more in human life is already within us and around us in the world; we are already, in some sense, participating in it. Hence transcendence (more) is also immanence. What we pay attention to or give care to is what is more . . . *we give it priority in our lives*, we are in *awe* of it: it is sacred to us. Insofar as we give priority in human life to what is more in human life than meets the eye, we desire to live and move *with* it, not against it.[45]

The term *Tantra* can refer to the vast Tāntric tradition in general, to particular subsystems of thought and practice, and to Tāntric texts. There are many classifications of the subtraditions of Tantra. Tantra may be Hindu or non-Hindu, that is, Buddhist or Jain. Five major divisions of Hindu Tantra, based on predomination of particular deities, are the Śakta, Śaiva, Saura, Gāṇapatya, and Vaiṣṇava, and there are other subdivisions within and besides these. Discussion here and in chapter 4 examines Tāntric approaches to body and religious therapeutics, at points referring to views of particular sub-traditions, but without intending them to be representative of the whole Tāntric tradition.

Tāntric texts are sometimes called *Āgamas*, but this term refers more specifically to the Śaiva texts.[46] The Āgama literature is extensive, but is more concerned with religious practice than with philosophical speculation.[47] An anti-ascetic and anti-speculative orientation is characteristic of Tantra. Although Tantra has comprehensive metaphysical foundations, it is mainly concerned with *sādhana*, religious practice. Hindu Tantra has philosophical contributions in addition to those of the six Veda-accepting classical *darśanas*, yet much of Tāntric philosophy involves modifications of Sāṃkhya and Vedānta.[48]

Tantra as a major religious and philosophical movement emerged around the fourth century of the common era. According to Eliade, Tantra "assumed the form of a pan-Indian vogue from the sixth century onward," popular among philosophers and theologians as well as ascetics and yogins, and influential in philosophy, mysticism, ritual, ethics, iconography, and literature.[49] The origins of Tantra are not precisely known, but in the pre-Vedic Indus Valley civilization, centuries before the common era, the germs of Tantra existed in the worship of the Mother Goddess, and the Mother and Father of the universe.[50] Tantra rejects the caste system and the exclusion of females from participation in religious activities. Tantra has long provided a religious domain for persons excluded from the Brahminical system because of caste or gender, as well as for those whose religious ideas and practice diverge from Hindu orthodoxy. Though Tāntrism is a major current of Indian culture, it has tended to remain on the fringes of society.[51] Tantra has been misunderstood—and maligned—for advocating activities that are traditionally or morally objectionable, and among the many subtraditions of Tantra, some do involve extreme and even bizarre practices. Ritual sexual union (both actual and symbolic) is an aspect of some forms of Tantra. However, to reduce the whole tradition of Tantra to particular sects or rites, or to reject Tantra based on a sensationalized view, would be a misconstrual of this vital aspect of Indian philosophy and religion.

Like the Vedic tradition, Tantra's foremost concern is spiritual realization, but its approach to the relation of human being, world, and the sacred aims for transcendence of materiality by *integration* with it, rather than separation from it. Liberation as conceived in Tantra includes spiritual well-being in this life. S. C. Banerji writes that "Tāntric philosophy vigorously advocates *jīvanmukti* (liberation in life)."[52] In comparing the "emancipative core" of psychoanalysis and Tantra, Sudhir Kakar writes that in Tantra, liberation is not only the "mystical" freedom from all human conditions, but is "also relevant to the individual's concrete historical conditions."[53] Tantra's soteriological goal is the realization of the unity of the individual's soul or *jīva* with the one Supreme Reality, *Param Śiva*, which has the static and transcendent aspect *Śiva*, and the dynamic and immanent aspect *Śakti*. The masculine *Śiva* is pure Being, of the nature of consciousness, and the feminine *Śakti* is the power that activates and manifests *Śiva*: "The universe is a manifestation of the immanent aspect of the *Parama Śiva* in the form of *Śakti*."[54] While *Śíva* is Being, *Śakti* is the *operative* form of Being, called in the *Yoginīhṛdaya*: 'the creative matrix' (*ṣṛṣtirūpā*).[55] *Śakti* and *Śiva* are one, as water and its current are one. A person could object to this analogy and the Tāntric ontology it illustrates, saying that the current is not essential to the water, but is a property of the water, or that the water needn't have a current, for it could be motionless. Tantra would reply that *Śakti* is the form and force of every manifestation of *Śiva:* roiling, trickling, or completely still, *Śakti* is the force responsible for the water's state. The word *Śakti* literally means power or energy [√ *śak*, 'to be able']. *Śiva* derives from the verbal root √ *śī*, 'to lie,' and connotes 'that in which all lies,' as well as meaning kind, gracious, and the like.

The *Mahānirvāṇa Tantra* begins with Parvatī (Śakti) the spouse of Śiva, asking him "What will lead to the benefit of the universe?" Śiva replies by conveying the nature of *Brahman*, the worship of whom leads to liberation.

> O Parameśvarī! Should good be done to the universe, the Lord of the universe is pleased, since he is its Self, and it depends on him. He is One. He ever is. He is the truth. He is supreme unity without a second. He is ever-full and self-manifest. He is eternal consciousness and bliss.
>
> MNT 1:33.3–4

About her own nature, Parvatī hears from Śiva:

> Thou art the very *Para Prakṛti* (supreme matter) of *Brahman* the *Paramātman* (supreme consciousness) and from thee has sprung the whole universe—O Śivā—its Mother. O gracious one, whatever is in this world, of things that have and are without motion, from *Mahat* (the Great) to an atom, owes its origin to and is dependent on thee. . . . Thou art both subtle and gross, manifested and veiled, though in Thyself formless, yet thou hast form.
>
> MNT 4:10–11, 15

Tāntric metaphysics include *prakṛti* and *puruṣa*, but they are understood differently from the way classical Yoga understands them. Yoga faces the general quandary of dualistic ontologies, that of explaining how two entities of wholly distinct natures can interact. According to Yoga, *puruṣa* is pure consciousness, and *prakṛti* is unconscious matter. There are many *puruṣas;* each person is an individual *puruṣa*. Tantra however, like Vedānta, accepts *Brahman* as the one real. According to Tantra, both the individual *puruṣa*, and *prakṛti* or material mature, are identical with *Brahman*. While Yoga holds that creation proceeds from the co-presence of *prakṛti* and *puruṣa*, in Tantra, both *prakṛti* and *puruṣa* exist within the supreme *Brahman*. Like Vedānta, Tantra considers creation to proceed from *līlā:* the sportive play of *Brahman*. Thus for Tantra, *prakṛti* is not distinct from *Brahman*, nor is *prakṛti* unconscious (*jaḍa*) as it is for Yoga. As part of *Brahman*, *prakṛti* is conscious, and by means of *prakṛti*, *Brahman* manifests itself in the form of all the constituents of the manifest universe.[56] Tantra's metaphysical presupposition that matter possesses consciousness is crucial: classical Yoga assumes that matter is unconscious, and aims for realization of Self as not-matter, but Tāntric yoga utilizes the body as an instrument of liberation, and reveres its material nature as both conscious and sacred.

While Tāntric metaphysics is non-dualistic (*advaitin*), and regards *Brahman*, known as *Param Śiva*, as the one Reality, it allows for the apparent difference of the one Absolute and the multifarious manifest world. Śiva and Śakti are separable in empirical and cognitive analysis, but their identity is knowable through higher knowledge offered by Tāntric mysticism.[57] Tantra is non-dualistic like Vedānta, rather than dualistic like Yoga, but while Vedānta ultimately relegates the manifest world to the status of *māyā* or illusion, Tantra considers the manifest world as fully real. Vedānta regards *māyā* as "that power (*Śakti*) of Brahman by which the world of multiplicity comes into existence."[58] Tantra shares this interpretation, but not Advaita Vedānta's understanding of *māyā* as the illusory ground and nature of subject-object distinctions.

> What is meant by calling the world an illusion and at the same time ascribing existence to it? The answer is that for Advaita Vedānta the term "real" means that which is permanent, eternal, infinite, that which is *trikālābādhyam*, never subrated at any time by another experience—and *Brahman* alone fits this meaning. The world is not real, but it is not wholly unreal.[59]

For Tantra however, material nature (including the embodied human being) is a manifestation of Śiva-Śakti, has full reality, and is sacred in its origin and fundamental nature. The human being as an aspect of creation is not-different from *Param Śiva*. This ontological position contributes to a more body-positive religious practice and soteriological goal than is found in orthodox Hinduism.

Tantra's monistic view of the world and *Brahman* (as Śiva-Śakti) is free of the metaphysical problems confronted by the dualism of classical Yoga. Further, even though Tantra is monistic, it is able, unlike Advaita Vedānta, to preserve the particularity of entities. Rather than ascribing to particular entities a lower ontological status as mere appearances of *Brahman* (a consequence of Advaita Vedānta's understanding of *māyā*) Tāntric metaphysics does not consider particular entities in the manifest world to be less real than *Brahman*. For persons who are concerned about provision for particularity, as is the case when body is considered integral to personhood, Tāntric metaphysics makes an important contribution. According to Tantra, not just the person's consciousness, but consciousness and the psychophysical complex together are *Brahman*. The body is the person's locus in space, and has a particular position and nature, with no less reality than the person's non-material aspects.

Reverence toward the beings and things of the world does not imply attachment and indulgence. Rather, Tantra considers recognition of the unity and sanctity of material nature as an antidote to attachment, for attachment requires a sense of duality. In the words of Kamalakar Mishra, "I can be attached [only] to something which I consider different from or other to me." By realizing that I am one with all, "there is no question of attachment with what is already myself or my own."[60] Eliade expresses the core of Tāntric metaphysics and soteriology as follows:

> . . . the absolute reality, the *Urgrund*, contains in itself all dualities and polarities, but reunited, reintegrated, in a state of absolute Unity (*advaya*). The creation, and the becoming that arose from it, represent the shattering of the primordial unity and the separation of the two principles (Śiva-Śakti, etc.); in consequence, man experiences a state of duality (object-subject, etc.)—and this is suffering, illusion, "bondage." The purpose of Tāntric *sādhana* is the reunion of the two polar principles within the disciple's own body.[61]

Consonant with other Indian traditions, Tantra holds that liberation depends on self-knowledge. The individual, or *jīva*, is Śiva, and Tāntric *sādhana* serves the purpose of gaining self-knowledge: *ātma-pratyabhijña*. Mishra names *pratyabhijña* ('recognition') as the central problem of the Tāntric tradition of Kaśmīra Śaivism. He notes that this school is in agreement with Advaita Vedānta on the point that self is known not as an object in a dualistic subject-object way, but is known as a self-illumined or *svayamprakāśa* subject.[62] Self-realization in Tantra is considered to afford both ultimate liberation and enjoyment in the present life.[63]

Classical Yoga envisions liberation as realization of Self-nature as pure consciousness, without suffering, but without bliss. Tantra, however, like Vedānta, conceives the liberated state as one of Being, consciousness, and bliss. However, in Tāntric practice, body is central in the quest for liberative self-knowledge.

A main tenet of Tāntric practice or *sādhana* is that "the Absolute is to be realized in and through the human body."[64] The universe is Śiva's manifestation, and the human body is Śiva's abode. The body is the quintessence of the physioconscious creation, and the Tāntric practitioner or *sādhaka* awakens the divinity within him- or herself with the orientation expressed in the *Ratnasāra Tantra* that "one who realizes the truth of the body can then come to know the truth of the universe."[65] Eliade writes that in Tāntrism, the body assumes an importance unparalleled in the Indian tradition:

> To be sure, health and strength, interest in a physiology homologizable with the cosmos and implicitly sanctified, are Vedic, if not pre-Vedic, values. But Tāntrism carries to its furthest consequences the conception that sanctity can be realized only in a "divine body." The Upaniṣadic and post-Upaniṣadic pessimism and asceticism are swept away. The body is no longer the source of pain, but the most reliable and effective instrument at man's disposal for "conquering death."[66]

Eliade distinguishes two convergent orientations in Tantra's valuation of the body:

1. Emphasis on *the total experience of life* as integral to Tāntric *sādhana*.
2. The will to master and transmute the body into a divine body, a strong theme in Haṭha Yoga.[67]

Central to Tantra is the polarity of macrocosm and microcosm, wherein the human body is realized—through the interiorization of ritual—as a microcosm of the universe. The language of 'macrocosm/microcosm' conveys Tantra's metaphysical orientation, but only in practice can one grasp the meaning of realizing oneself, in body and consciousness, as being part of the whole seamless conscious creation. Although writers on Tantra use the terminology of macrocosm/microcosm, it would be more consonant with Tāntric metaphysics to speak in terms of *correspondence* throughout the domains of being. Tāntric unity of self and cosmos is a variant of Vedic macranthropy. The *Atharva-veda,* for instance, identifies the breaths with the cosmic winds [AV 11: 4.15]. The *Upaniṣads* contain references to the identification of the breath with the cardinal directions [Chānd. Up. 3:13.1–6]. While air "weaves the universe" [Bṛhad Up. 3:7.2], breath "weaves" the human being [AV 10:2.13]. The spinal column is equated with the world-axis Mount Meru in the Tāntric text *Dohakoṣa*. The *iḍā-naḍī* and *piṅgalā-naḍī* (corresponding with the two principal breaths *prāṇa* and *apāna)* are called sun and moon, symbolizing their respective strong and gentle natures.[68] Tāntric practice or *sādhana* utilizes cosmophysiology to transubstantiate the human being, to sanctify the human being by practices that 'dilate' or 'cosmicize' the physical body so the practitioner realizes her- or himself as literally one with the Absolute that forms the whole of nature—physical and conscious.

Purity—physical and religious—is a major concern in Hinduism. Tantra reevaluates the meaning of impurity, and recasts traditional associations between physical impurity and unholiness. A significant example is that Tantra rejects the notion that the touch of a low-caste person would make something impure. The equating of physical impurity with religious impurity is rejected as well. For instance, body fluids are considered by Tantra as physically unclean, but not unholy.[69] Tantra operates on the principle that all aspects of the world, and particularly those of the human psychophysical complex, are to be accepted and sublimated.[70] The word 'sublimate' derives from the Latin *sublīmāre* 'to raise,' [*sublīmus*, 'uplifted,' 'sublime'].[71] In the Tāntric context, *sublimate* pertains to raising the cruder physical level of being to its real status as divine. Renunciation in Tantra does not mean asceticism, but "proper utilization of an object."[72] Contemporary Indian scholars and practitioners of Tantra acknowledge that Tantra is subject to criticism because of the actions of "hypocrites and pseudo-tāntrists," who "actually worship their own ego and gratify their senses and do nothing else."[73] Sensationalized stereotypes are put into perspective in chapter 4's discussion of Tāntric utilization of life energy, including the sexual force, for spiritual attainment.

Body as the Ground of Well-being in Āyurveda

Āyurveda is called "a principal architect of the Indian view of person and body" by psychoanalyst Sudhir Kakar.[74] His fieldwork investigating India's healing traditions demonstrates that in some significant ways, Āyurveda's approach to the body diverges from traditional religio-philosophical views. Although Yoga is well known for supporting the health of body, Āyurveda is actually the Indian *śāstra* or discipline directly concerned with health and healing. The word *Āyurveda* is composed of *āyus*, 'life,' and *veda*, 'knowledge.' Āyurveda means knowledge of life and longevity, and designates a system of healthful living based on knowledge. For personal health maintenance, Āyurveda makes recommendations emphasizing diet, cleansing and rejuvenative measures, and daily and seasonal regimen. As a system of medicine, Āyurveda has eight branches and is thus called *aṣṭāṅga* (eight-limbed) *Āyurveda*.

The Eight Branches of Āyurvedic Medicine

1. Internal medicine, including physiology and pathology: *Kāya-cikitsā*
2. General surgery: *Śalyāpahartṛka*
3. Eye, ear, nose and throat disease: *Śālākya*
4. Pediatrics, including obstetrics and embryology: *Kaumāra bhṛtya*
5. Psychology/psychiatry: psychotherapy, dream analysis, demonology: *Bhūta-vidyā*
6. Toxicology: *viśagara-vairodhika-praśamana*
7. Geriatrics: and rejuvenation therapy: *Rasāyana*
8. Sexology: *Vājikaraṇa* [75]

Body and physical health and illness are central in Āyurvedic medicine. While body and health are important in classical Yoga, Yoga has *consciousness* as its primary subject and agent of liberation. Yoga and Āyurveda are sister sciences: practitioners of Yoga may study Āyurveda prior to and along with their practice of Yoga, and Āyurveda's science of the body serves to make the body more fit and pure for undertaking the spiritual science of Yoga. Moreover, when yogic disciplines are performed, the activation of stagnant energies in the body/mind may result in physical and psychological disorders that can be diagnosed and treated with Āyurvedic methods.[76]

Yoga and Āyurveda have in common strongly (but not exclusively) Sāṃkhya metaphysical foundations, and in many respects their theory and practice constitute applications of Sāṃkhya principles. A major difference between Āyurveda and Yoga is that Āyurveda is primarily directed toward the earthly goals of health and longevity, while Yoga has spiritual liberation as its aim. Āyurveda is not, however, without religious roots and applications. Its ultimate source is Brahmā the creator, who gave the knowledge of Āyurveda through the *ṛṣis* or seers who produced the divinely intuited Vedas. Āyurveda's claim to divine origin grounds its assertion that it is not limited to any particular culture, religion, or period of history. As a source of knowledge it considers itself to have no beginning or end: Āyurveda deals with things inherent in nature, and based on the assumption that such natural manifestations are eternal, the principles regarding medicine and health remain constant, though in application their concrete particulars differ [CS 1:30.27]. Yoga is a liberative discipline, a *mokṣa-śāstra* whose benefits are also germane across time, place, and circumstances. Though Āyurveda is not a *mokṣa-śāstra,* the

Caraka-saṃhitā states that Āyurveda is sacred because it benefits humankind in "both worlds," this one, and the life beyond [CS 1:1.43].

The Āyurvedic texts present medical theory in the context of medical *practice*, so the theoretical principles of Āyurveda have to be pieced together and conceptually reconstructed. Jean Filliozat writes that Āyurvedic medicine is a rational system based on experience, and Gerald Larson corroborates this by describing the practical operational character of the medical literature, wherein symptoms and diseases are classified, contextualized with respect to diagnosis, prognosis, and so on, then addressed therapeutically.[77] The major texts that have preserved knowledge of Āyurveda to the present day are together called *Bṛhattrayi*, "The Great Trio." The encyclopedic *Caraka-saṃhitā*, compiled in the first centuries of the common era, and commented on and revised in subsequent centuries, is used in present-day traditional Indian medical practice. The *saṃhitā* or collection of Suśruta is similar in content to the *saṃhitā* of Caraka, except that the *Suśruta-saṃhitā* emphasizes surgery.[78] The third major Āyurvedic text is the *Aṣṭāṅga-hṛdaya-saṃhitā* of Vagbhata.[79]

The *Caraka-saṃhitā* has eight volumes. Its chapters deal with concerns of practical medicine such as pathogenesis, diagnosis, pharmaceuticals, and therapeutic measures. The first volume, *Sūtra-sthāna* ('the section on fundamentals'), presents essential principles of maintaining health and preventing and curing disease; thus it is particularly valuable for study of Āyurveda's concepts of health and the philosophical and religious implications of Āyurvedic medical philosophy.

Caraka describes Āyurveda as "the science through the knowledge of which one can obtain knowledge about the useful and harmful types of life, happy and miserable types of life, things that are useful for such types of life, the span of life and the very nature of life" [CS 1:1.41]. Āyurveda's aim is preservation and restoration of health, and assistance in attaining the four *puruṣārthas* or principles of life: *dharma* (righteousness), *artha* (prosperity), *kāma* (enjoyment), and *mokṣa* (liberation) [CS 1:1.15]. Āyurveda's commitment to the *puruṣārthas* demonstrates that Āyurveda serves the quest for religious liberation and is not merely for material well-being.

The origins of Āyurveda are evident in the *Atharva-veda* (c. 1500–1000 B.C.E.), in which both religious (e.g., māntric), and medical (e.g., pharmacological) approaches to healing are represented. Hundreds of medicinal plants are listed in the Vedas, as, for instance, in this passage:

> Most efficacious for healing this disease [leprosy] is the medicine known as Rajanī, thou posessest the healing power of Suparna. Asuri-named

> medicine lends its color and shape to different plants, and is made serviceable through pulverization.
>
> AV 1:5.24.1

Rajanī (√ *rañj*, 'to color') refers to the medicinal plant turmeric: *Curcuma Longa*. It is generally called *Haridrā* in the *Caraka-saṃhita*. Following is an example of a māntric or prayer approach to healing:

> O maladies, whether ye result from physical or ancestral ailments, or the company of ignoble persons, or are sprung out of cherishing evil thoughts, get ye away from here.
>
> AV 1:3.14.5

Prayers or incantations—often incorporating images of nature, as is characteristic of Vedic texts—may accompany medical procedures, such as a surgeon's opening a patient's obstructed urinary passage:

> Just as the pent-up water of a lake is let loose by cleaving its dam, so do I, O patient open thy urinary passage. May that urine of thine come out completely, free from check.
>
> AV 1:1.3.7

Environmental factors are not merely metaphoric, but are important in Vedic etiology and therapeutics, as evident in this prayer for the physician's success:

> O physician, so thou release this man from headache, free him from cough which has entered into all his limbs and joints. One should resort to forests and hills for relief from diseases resulting from excessive rains, severe wind and intense heat.
>
> AV 1:3.12.3

Āyurvedic medicine abandons the ancient Vedic religio-magical therapeutics. However, the role of the environment in the cause and cure of illness remains central. Francis Zimmermann's study of Āyurveda, *The Jungle and the Aroma of Meats: An Ecological Theme in Hindu Medicine*, presents Āyurveda as grounded in ecological theory that conceives of the land and the human body as the two kinds of place. Prognosis was informed by knowledge of the influences of climate, season, diet, and custom. Therapeutic intervention had the double purpose of:

1. Rendering the environment appropriate to the needs of the patient (by relocating the patient to a climate suitable to his constitution and malady).

2. Rendering the patient's diet and regimen appropriate to the ecological conditions.

While ancient Greco-Latin science produced the model of knowledge called natural history, based on classification of species according to empirically grounded distinctions, the concern of Indian taxonomy was the dietetic and therapeutic qualities of the land and its inhabitants. Āyurveda's concept of the person places the human being within a context of 'biogeography,' an aspect of the broader register of knowledge called pharmacy. Pharmacy presupposes a whole cosmic physiology: the great chain of foods where living beings—eaters and eaten—transmit to one another the nourishing essences of the soil. Pharmacy then leads to a superior register of knowledge: physiology, which in the ancient sense embraces

> . . . the circulation of fluids in the surrounding world, the rise of sap in plants, the aroma that is given off by the cooking of different kinds of meats, and finally the interplay of different humors within the body.[80]

While Āyurveda utilizes concepts of the person based to a great extent on Sāṃkhya and Vaiṣeśika metaphysics, the person as the subject of medical science is regarded within a context of the web of life. Āyurveda as 'knowledge of life' refers not just to individual human life, but to the whole of living nature, and the countless pathogenic and therapeutic factors influencing human health.

'Life' in the context of individual health-maintenance embraces more than biological life sustained by medical science. Āyurveda provides a system of hygiene incorporating such factors as diet and seasonal regimen, cleanliness and physical purification, and cultivation of knowledge and attitudes that sustain well-being. Knowledge of *life* in Āyurveda strongly concerns hygiene (Gk. *hygienos:* 'healthful'), the study and practice of preserving health and preventing illness. Compared with the dramatic achievements of medical science, the idea of hygiene as a significant part of health-care is often considered to be on the level of archaic folk remedies. Āyurveda's systematic and sophisticated theory of hygiene counters such a view. Granted, contemporary scientific medicine makes remarkable contributions to human well-being, but hygiene remains foundational to health, and the power of medical science to prevent and treat medical problems doesn't replace the simple procedures of protecting and cultivating one's vitality. Furthermore, scientific medicine is concerned primarily with disease, and its theoretical basis gives insufficient attention to promoting health as a positive state.

Hygiene in the Āyurvedic sense of 'knowledge of life' is the axis of the ancient medical traditions of Greece and China as well as India. Although these medical systems developed advanced medical knowledge and procedures, the foundation of each was proper hygienic measures. Plato's *Timaeus* says of diseases:

> . . . if anyone regardless of the appointed time tries to subdue them by medicine, he only aggravates and multiplies them. Wherefore we ought always to manage them by regimen, as far as a man can spare the time, and not provoke a disagreeable enemy by medicines.[81]

The *Huang Ti Nei Ching Su Wên,* "The Yellow Emperor's Classic of Internal Medicine," opens with discussion of why people become so decrepit and no longer live to be a hundred years old. The answer: formerly, they practiced temperance based on understanding the *tao* and conducted themselves in accord with *yin* and *yang.*

> There was temperance in eating and drinking. Their hours of rising and retiring were regular and not disorderly and wild. By these means the ancients kept their bodies united with their souls, so as to fulfil their allotted span completely, measuring unto a hundred years before they passed away.[82]

The *Caraka-saṃhitā*—along with its extensive presentation of theory and procedures for prevention, diagnosis, and treatment by pharmacological, surgical, and other means—conveys many points of hygiene, such as recommendations for diet, exercise, seasonal regimen, grooming, massage, and maintaining the physique. Cakrapāṇidatta's commentary, *Āyurveda Dīpikā,* states that "of all the factors for the maintenance of positive health, food taken in proper quantity occupies the most important position" [AD 1:5.1]. Several verses are devoted to instruction on the taking and healthful utilization of nourishment. For instance, it is recommended that one note the relative heaviness of food, and leave about one-third of one's stomach capacity unfilled, to assist the power of digestion [CS 1:5.7]. In the humble matter of consuming food, Āyurveda reveals a serious implication of the ancient medical systems' emphasis on 'knowledge of life': the individual's self-responsibility and power to maintain his or her own health. Āyurveda emphasizes:

1. The individual's particular type of constitution—physical and psychological.
2. A holistic theory of the environment, focusing on the individual's

relationship with the environment in the diagnosis and treatment of health problems.

3. Concepts of health and disease that incorporate interrelated dimensions of human physiology, psychology, and spirituality.
4. Sustaining health as a positive state.
5. Prevention of health problems.

The Āyurvedic texts have a strongly Sāṃkhyan account of the nature of person and body (evident in passages such as *Caraka-saṃhitā* IV:1, *Suśruta-saṃhitā* III). Life arises from the co-presence of consciousness and primordial materiality. Materiality operates through the interaction of the three energy-forces called *guṇas* ('strands' or 'ropes'). Larson characterizes the *guṇas* as follows: *sattva,* the subtle matter of pure thought, *rajas,* the kinetic matter of pure energy, and *tamas,* the reified matter of inertia.[83] All forms of matter, including the human body and senses, are composed at a fundamental level of the five *mahābhūtas* or subtle elements (space, air, fire, water, and earth), each produced by a particular combination of the *guṇas*. The five *mahābhūtas* in turn combine to form the three *dhātus* or *doṣas* that constitute the psychophysical person (see Figure 1.1). Along with drawing on Sāṃkhya as a dominant philosophical basis, Āyurveda also uses terms and concepts from other Veda-accepting systems—Nyāya, Vaiṣeśika, Vedānta, and Yoga—as well as from the non-Vedic systems Buddhism and Jainism. Mainly Nyāya, Vaiṣeśika, and Buddhist theories explain physical and chemical processes in Āyurveda, while Sāṃkhya is considered to provide a very adequate metaphysics and account of the process of creation.[84] Larson suggests that the affinity between Āyurveda and the naturalistic philosophical systems generated a mutually influential pattern of interaction. The meaning of *darśana,* 'viewpoint,' as the designation of the major Indian philosophical systems—considered as complementary and non-contradictory despite the differences of their principles and methods—is wonderfully exemplified by Āyurveda's employment of these several systems.

Sāṃkhya metaphysics grounds the central doctrine of Āyurvedic metaphysiology, that of the *dhātus* (*doṣas*) or constitutive principles of human psychophysiology and pathology. The three *guṇas* produce the five subtle proto-elements or *mahābhūtas,* and the proto-elements combine in three pairs to form the body's three *dhātus,* fundamental elements or 'supports' (√ *dhā,*'to give,' e.g., 'to give support').

Āyurveda uses the term *dhātu* in two ways. First, the body is held to have seven *dhātus* or basic tissue elements, each derived from the one preceding it in the following sequence: *rasa* (chyle or extract of nutriment),

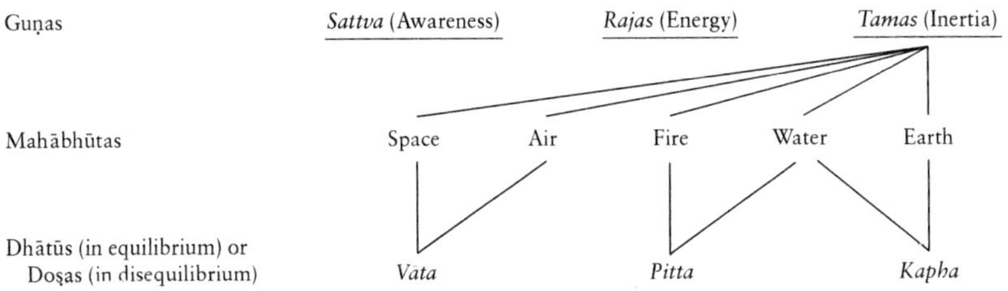

Figure 1.1 Āyurveda's three *dhātus* or *doṣas*

blood, flesh, fat, bone, marrow, and ova/semen. The term *dhātu* also refers to the three functional constituents of the body/mind: *vāta, pitta, and kapha*. In a normal and healthy state these three function in dynamic equilibrium and are called *dhātus*. When one or more of the three *dhātus* is aggravated or diminished, equilibrium is compromised and they are called *doṣas* (√ *duṣ*: 'to spoil,' 'to impair'. The term *tri-doṣa* signifies the three 'faults' or 'impairments' that condition disease.

A major manifestation of the three *doṣas* is the body's systems of respiration (*vata*), digestion (*pitta*), and structural integration (*kapha*). Each *doṣa* has characteristic functions within the body. *Vāta* is the dynamic element in digestion, excretion, respiration, circulation, reproductive functions, speech, and motor activity in general. *Pitta* is the energy of the vision, the nervous system, and the digestive 'cooking' of food in the stomach. *Kapha* is responsible for the integration of tissues and systems, and maintenance of the body's homeostasis. *Vāta, pitta,* and *kapha* are generally translated as 'wind,' 'bile,' and 'phlegm,' but instead of taking these terms literally, they should be understood as the principles constituting and governing the body's systems and functions.

Āyurveda's practice of health-care assumes a concept of the person as a 'tripod' of body, mind, and self, which together constitute the sentient 'person' called *puruṣa* [CS 1:1.46–47]. The tripod metaphor suggests that these three constituents serve as a substratum to support the person's higher nature, but it is the tripod that is Āyurveda's practical subject matter. Human life, according to this rather Vaiṣeśikan interpretation in the *Caraka-saṃhitā,* arises from the association of the body, *śarīra* (including its sensory capacities), with the mind *(sattva* or *manas*), and self (*ātman*). This association constitutes the person who is of concern to Āyurveda.

While Yoga regards the person's ultimate nature as *puruṣa* or pure consciousness, and its aim is the freeing of this spiritual Self from the body, Āyurveda inclines toward the cooperation of the physical and the spiritual. Cromwell Crawford comments that "for Āyurveda, spirit and matter, soul and body, although different, are not alien, insofar as they can be brought in a healing relationship with consequences that are mutually beneficial."[85] Āyurveda thus diverges from the position of classical Sāṃkhya and Yoga that consciousness should transcend materiality. This is a central example of how Āyurveda, because it is concerned with concrete physical problems, embodies and reveals meanings about human nature that deviate from traditional Indian religious and textual interpretations.

Although Āyurveda does not draw the same soteriological conclusions from Sāṃkhya cosmology that Yoga does, the Sāṃkhya philosophy of cosmic evolution is part of the foundation of Āyurveda's conception of the human being as a microcosm within the macrocosm of the natural world. Crawford articulates the point that the "parallelism between human nature and nature at large suggests that humans are in a systemic relationship with the creative forces of the universe."[86] This point is illuminated by Zimmermann's analysis of Āyurveda's doctrine of humors and the medical formulation of a cosmic physiology dominated by the themes of the circulation of fluids and the chain of successive 'cookings' of nutriment by the sun, the cooking fire, and the digestion. The Āyurvedic version of the great chain of Being is a chain of foods, where essences transmitted from the soils, through plants, herbivores, carnivores, and man are finally rendered to the gods in the aroma of sacrificial fires. The burning transformative power of the sun, the cooking fire, the digestive fire, metabolism, and the flames of sacrifice are links in a universe of biospiritual metamorphosis, where the meal is a metaphoric ritualization of sacrificing foods in the internal fire.[87]

Caraka's text *Analysis of the Human Body* reveals Āyurveda's conception of the body in a more fundamental way than the accounts given in the *Caraka-saṃhitā*. The text does not address anatomy and physiology conceived in terms of the structure and function of the body's organs and systems. According to Zimmermann, Caraka's *Analysis of the Human Body* is "a speculative pathogenesis, a reflection of balance and imbalance between the humors from which results either growth or wasting of the tissues."[88] Caraka's text begins with a definition of the body as *samyogavahin*, translated by Zimmermann as "a vehicle for congruous junctions." The physician's work is to orchestrate proper conjunctions of foods and medicinal substances with the patient's particular constitution and circumstances—environmental and temporal as well as pathological. The next chapter, "Meanings of Health in Āyurveda," presents a set of determinants of health based on Hindu medicine's holistic conception of person and world.

Chapter Two

MEANINGS OF HEALTH IN ĀYURVEDA

In Western philosophy of medicine, inquiries into health tend to focus more on the meanings of disease, in part because disease demands concrete problem-solving for a variety of ills, while health is assumed to be a unitary state equivalent to the absence of disease or dysfunction. This chapter examines the notion of health as a positive state, rejecting the narrow definition that health is simply the absence of disease. Contemporary scientific medicine is oriented to treating specific syndromes to the neglect of addressing the well-being of the whole person. This approach to health and healing is being questioned by many patients and practitioners.[1] Ancient and traditional health-care systems—such as India's Āyurveda—have roots in religious cosmologies that regard the person as more than body or body/mind, but as inclusive of a spiritual dimension, and as part of the natural world and the social world. An Āyurvedic understanding of 'medicine' incorporates not just pharmacology, surgery, and the other empirical disciplines we associate with the word. The close relation of medicine and religion is reflected in the etymological fact that the Indo-European root *med*, 'to take appropriate measures,' is the source of the words 'medicine' and 'meditation.' Among *med's* descendents are the Latin *mederī*, 'to look after,' and *meditārī* 'to think about.'

Traditional healing systems can broaden our views of the nature of the person, and of religious, social, and environmental implications of health and illness. They can also open perspectives for a more comprehensive understanding of health. The commonality of medicine and religion—at root, the perpetuation of human well-being—underlies concern for both psychophysical and spiritual health in traditions across lands and times. While Āyurveda has much to offer as a system of medicine and as a program of health maintenance, my task here is not to evaluate the soundness of Āyurvedic medical theory. Rather, I follow Gerald Larson's suggestion that South Asian medical theory and practice can reveal new agendas for health and healing.

> What is of importance in traditional medicine, however, is a way of valuing and a way of conceptualizing "disease" and "illness" that is interestingly different from our own and that is not at all incompatible with the rigorous precision of modern scientific methodology.[2]

A foundational concept of Āyurvedic medical philosophy is *equilibrium*, starting with the idea of health as balance among the three *doṣas* or bioenergetic principles. The idea of balance has a range of applications, such as a suitable ratio of work, rest, and recreation, and the eating of types and amounts of food in proportion to individual requirements and digestive capacity. Āyurveda's fourfold therapeutic paradigm is given in *Caraka-saṃhitā* 1:9.19, shown below.

The Four Branches of Āyurvedic Medical Knowledge

1. Causes of diseases
2. Diagnosis
3. Cure
4. Prevention

This chapter presents a set of determinants of health, derived from the classical Āyurvedic text, Agniveśa's *Caraka-saṃhitā* (c. first century C.E.), and its commentary *Āyurveda-dīpikā* of Cakrapaṇidatta. In about the third century C.E., the text was reconstructed and annotated by Caraka (an individual or perhaps a school), and the name Caraka still designates it. In the eigth century, the redactor D ṛḍhabala again reconstituted and refined the *Caraka-saṃhitā*. Cakrapaṇidatta's commentary *Āyurveda-dīpikā* was written in the eleventh century.[3] Interpretive sources for this chapter include contemporary sources on Āyurveda, and modern Western medical philosophy. The purposes of this chapter are:

1. To offer a positive account of health applicable to human life in all its dimensions.
2. To specify major conditions of health in order to ground the idea of religious therapeutics.

Determinants of health are presented here under four categories:

1. Biological and ecological
2. Medical and psychological
3. Sociocultural and aesthetic
4. Metaphysical and religious

The four categories, and the determinants of health presented within them, are not intended to be entirely independent of one another, nor exhaustive.

INQUIRY INTO HEALTH

'Health' pertains to a state of being, but it also names a conceptual rubric, encompassing themes such as freedom from incapacitation, vitality sufficient for successful action, and feelings of well-being. 'Health-care' is a related rubric covering traditional and contemporary systems of medicine, preventive routines and treatment methods, and social issues such as the economics of health insurance. What we call 'health-care' in contemporary scientific medicine more often amounts to 'sickness care,' in that medical intervention is more often applied after illness has developed, rather than beforehand to cultivate the person's inherent vitality and to diagnose and prevent potential problems. Āyurveda emphasizes preventive methods and cultivation of health as a positive state, and provides a complement to the more crisis-oriented biomedical model. While the biomedical model gives most of its attention to the theory and treatment of disease, Āyurveda shows more concern for the active cultivation of health. Health is defined as follows in the preamble to the Constitution of the World Health Organization:

> Health is a state of complete physical, mental, and social well-being and not merely the absence of disease or infirmity.[4]

This definition has the strengths of recognizing the several domains of human life in which health is important, and of regarding health as a positive state, not merely a concept whose meaning is established in relation to illness or disability. Complete well-being or perfect health is generally thought to be an unrealizable ideal. We tend to think of healthiness as a matter of degree, for the complex web of relations among material and biological factors seems to obviate the possibility of the body's perfect form and function. Each of us, writes Susan Sontag in *Illness as Metaphor*, "holds dual citizenship, in the kingdom of the well and in the kingdom of the sick."[5] Yet perfect health is an ideal that physician Deepak

Chopra extends as possible through Āyurveda. Working from the Vedic premise that intelligence is the basic force underlying all of nature, Chopra's efforts to help restore Āyurveda in contemporary health-care invoke the Indian concept of the supreme Self (*Paramātman),* which Āyurveda says is free of dysfunction: "The soul is essentially devoid of abnormalities. . . . is eternal and the observer who sees all actions" [CS 1:1.56]. Chopra writes:

> There exists in every person a place that is free from disease, that never feels pain, that cannot age or die. When you go to this place, limitations that all of us accept cease to exist.[6]

Chopra explains Āyurveda's recommendations for a range of traditional practices of Āyurvedic physical culture, infused with the mental cultivation of meditation and the waking of body/mind intelligence. The "quantum mechanical body" is Chopra's model of a body of intelligence, which unites the 'river' of quanta comprising the physical body, with the 'river' of thought that is the mind.[7] Healing in quantum terms is grounded in knowledge (notably knowledge of oneself as a body of intelligence), and utilizes meditation and mental techniques "to control the invisible patterns that order the body."[8] Perfect health may not be possible, but the notion of it calls us to question what health could be like ideally. Āyurveda offers practical means of caring for one's body/mind that can help us live with more vitality, calmness, and well-being than we might have imagined.

In clarifying meanings concerning the relation of health and illness, it is worthwhile to acknowledge the ambiguities that make health and illness poles in a dialectical tension where one or the other may predominate. Our participation in the kingdom of the sick and the kingdom of the well is not as simple as occupying one realm and then the other. Conditions of sickness impinge to greater or lesser extents on states of health, and they even serve to mobilize the forces of health. The presence of disease or disability does not exclude health. As Caroline Whitbeck says, "a high degree of health is compatible with some degree of disease, injury, or impairment."[9] The "ambiguity of life" is Paul Tillich's term for the source of inevitable intrusions by destructive factors that cause illness and injury. In Tillich's view of the dialectic processes that constitute life, every creative process implies a destructive trend, and every integrating process implies a disintegrating trend. Threats exist even in the assimilation of food, breath, and communication. Intrusion of destructive forces, and thus malfunctions—physical and psychological—are inevitable. Disease, Tillich says, "is a symptom of the universal ambiguity of life."[10] In presenting determinants of health, I note ambiguities inherent in various aspects of health, and point out some of the tensions inherent in embodied human life as revealed through the window of health. An instance of such ambiguity is Nietzsche's startling suggestion that our seeking health without any sickness is cowardice, if not barbarism, for "the sick soul" as much as the healthy one, is needed to inspire self-knowledge and even virtue.[11] Nietzsche's recognition of the ambiguities inherent in human life and health suggests a useful direction for inquiry into the meaning of health: an adequate account of human health should allow for the fundamental tensions, ambiguities, and imperfections in human life.

Health and disease are not symmetrical concepts; that is, the meaning of one cannot be adequately established in terms of the other. H. Tristam Engelhardt holds that the concept of disease is a *pragmatic* concept, a concept by which phenomena are analyzed for the purposes of diagnosis, prognosis, and therapy. Health, on the other hand, is a *regulative* concept, a concept that establishes an ideal and guides inquiry and action toward the achievement of that ideal.[12] The Constitution of the World Health Organization provides an articulation of health as a regulative ideal, and it affirms health as a fundamental value for both the individual and for world culture:

- The enjoyment of the highest attainable standard of health is one of the fundamental rights of every human being without distinction of race, religion, political belief, economic or social condition.
- The health of all peoples is fundamental to the attainment of peace and security and is dependent upon the fullest co-operation of individuals and States.
- The achievement of any State in the promotion and protection of health is of value to all.[13]

Two influential doctrines of health illustrate descriptive and normative concepts of health. A *biologically based doctrine* articulated by Christopher Boorse defines health as "functional normality." This doctrine uses the terms 'health' and 'disease' as *descriptive*, value-neutral terms. To say that a person or an organ or system is healthy means that its functions are normal; to say it is diseased means that its functions are abnormal, with biostatistical data providing the criteria of normality.

> . . . diseases are internal states that depress a functional ability below species-typical levels. Health as freedom from disease is then statistical normality of function, i.e., the ability to perform all typical physiological functions with at least typical efficiency.[14]

Health and disease on this interpretation are employed as scientific concepts, not normative ones, despite the fact that, in general, human beings value health and abhor disease.

A *normative doctrine* is exemplified in Georg Canguilhem's *The Normal and the Pathological*, which uses the terms 'health' and 'disease' as *normative* terms: Health means that a person functions well, disease means he or she functions badly.

> Man feels in good health—what is health itself—only when he feels more than normal—that is, adapted to the environment and its demands—but normative, capable of following new norms of life. . . . for man health is a feeling of assurance in life to which no limit is fixed. *Valere*, from which value derives, means to be in good health in Latin. Health is a way of tackling existence as one feels that one is not only possessor or bearer but also, if necessary, creator of value, establisher of vital norms.[15]

Discussions of human health often address a particular dimension of health and neglect others, for instance, emphasizing the capacity to achieve one's goals but overlooking the factor of resistance to disease. Rather than proposing a 'definition' of health, I present a range of determinants that can be used as criteria for evaluating states of health, and that identify conditions for thinking about health. In using these determinants as criteria to assess the health of a particular person, emphasis may be placed on some determinants over others, depending on circumstances. For example, in evaluating the health of a child who has no serious medical problems, growth and development are important criteria of health. In the case of an elderly person with a chronic condition, the degree of pain experienced by the person would be a significant criterion. The determinants of health presented here are applicable across a range of instances, with modifications for specific circumstances. For example, strength is a criterion of health for both a child and an elderly person, though there are differences in the particular set of abilities required by each.

DETERMINANTS OF HEALTH

Biological and Ecological Determinants

Life, Development, and Longevity

Living, rather than dying, is a fundamental determinant of health. Health can be ascribed only of living entities, and an essential criterion of health is the organism's prevailing in its life-functions rather than tending toward death. Longevity means long life, and connotes living to great age with vitality. In Hindu medicine, life and longevity are central in the concept of health: *Āyurveda* means 'knowledge of life and longevity' (*āyus*, 'life'; *veda*, 'knowledge'). *Āyus* in the term Āyurveda means the combination of body, senses, mind, and soul [CS 1:1.42], but in the compound term *Āyurveda, āyus* connotes the support and prolonging of healthful human life [CS 1:1.41]. In Āyurveda, life means not merely biological thriving: the desire to live long and well is recommended as the first priority [CS 1:11.3–4].

The term 'development' applies to biological growth, but also to intellectual, social, and other kinds of progress in one's awareness and capabilities. Because human beings have high potential for intellectual, social, athletic, creative, and spiritual achievement, part of being healthy means cultivating one's knowledge and abilities. Without such lifelong development, a person tends more toward stagnation than toward optimum health. *Change* is an explanatory principle of the processes of life and development, and of disease and death as well. In biological terms, children's growth and development constitute change in the direction of healthiness, while impaired development marks problems with health, owing to factors such as inadequate nutrition, congenital abnormality, injury, or illness. Nineteenth-century pathologist Rudolph Virchow regarded diseases not as ontological entities, but as representing "the course of corporeal appearances under changed conditions."[16] Illness is marked by changes in sensations, capacities, and sometimes of appearance.[17] Change is integral to healing as well: to undergo healing is to undergo transformations wherein the normal conditions of life are restored, and to cure is to generate and assist transformations that restore the normal conditions of life.

Along with conception, death is an ultimate change of state of the physical body. Disease and injury may lead to death, yet there is such a thing as a 'healthy death,' a death experienced as part of the natural cycle of coming to be and passing away. Healthy death is exemplified by death from old age, when a person is not suffering greatly from the debilitation or pain of a particular condition. Instead, he or she retains a degree of strength and self-sufficiency until the time that the body has aged to the point that one or more systems cease to function. Āyurveda's notion of longevity means more than long life; it means cultivating long life in health and vitality, thus establishing conditions for a healthy death. At any age, the idea of 'healthy death' applies to cases where a person's powers to thrive are diminished, yet death is accepted with equanimity. The

Taoist idea of enlightenment as living and dying in accord with nature's simplicity grounds the notion of healthy death. Chuang Tzu rejected his disciples' plans for his funeral, named heaven and earth as his coffin, and accepted his imminent death without dread.[18] Poems by Zen Buddhist monks, written close to the moment of death, epitomize the idea of dying in a state of health sufficient to permit awareness and expression of one's final experience.[19]

Equilibrium

In Āyurveda the meaning of health centers on the concept of *equilibrium*. Healing involves restoration of balanced states of being within the organism—that is, at the level of the *doṣas* or constituent principles of the mind/body complex, and between organism and environment. Broadly conceived, equilibrium in Āyurveda means the stable and harmonious functioning of "our organs and systems, psyche and spirit, but also a balanced and creative relationship with our fellow creatures and nature as a whole."[20]

> The body and mind constitute the substrata of diseases and happiness (i.e., positive health). Balanced utilization (of time, mental faculties, and objects of sense organs) is the cause of happiness.
>
> CS 1:1.55

The technical meaning of equilibrium or balance in Āyurveda refers to the equilibrium of the three *dhātus* or *doṣas*. Health on the Āyurvedic interpretation is the equilibrium of *vāta*, *pitta*, and *kapha*, the *tri-dhātu*, the three 'tissue-elements,' more precisely termed 'systematic constituents' or 'sustaining factors.' Their imbalance constitutes impaired health, and is referred to as *tridoṣa*, the three systematic problems.

> The very object of this science is the maintenance of the equilibrium of the tissue elements [*dhātusāmya:* equilibrium of sustaining and nourishing factors].
>
> CS 1:1.53

> As the author himself will say, the disturbance of the equilibrium of tissue elements [*dhātus*] is the disease, while the maintenance of equilibrium is health.
>
> AD 1:1.53

Applications of *tridoṣa* theory include:

1. Classification of the patient's psychophysical constitution-type, determined by the predominance of one or more *doṣas*.

2. Etiological theory employing the explanatory principle of deviation from the proper proportions of the *doṣas*.
3. Therapeutic measures including pharmaceuticals that act to restore the balance of the *doṣas* according to the patient's constitutional type and environmental circumstances.

> For the maintenance of health, it is necessary that a perfect equilibrium be established with regard to the various forces acting and counteracting on the body. If there is an excessive deficiency anywhere, it has got to be neutralized. . . . Marshy lands are by nature dominated by the qualities of unctuousness ['oiliness,' 'slipperiness'] and heaviness. Individuals residing in such places should naturally be required to become used to taking meat of animals of arid climate, honey, etc., which are dominated by qualities like roughness and lightness in contradistinction with those of the unctuousness and heaviness which dominate the climate of other lands. Similarly, one should be required to follow a regular regimen on the above lines in order to counteract the imbalancing forces of these places. The same principle also holds good with regard to the various diseases. For example, if a disease has occurred due to the vitiation [impairment] of *vāta*, then the diet, drugs and regimen are to be habituated in such a manner that they counteract the effect of the former.
>
> AD 1:6.50

Āyurvedic physician Vasant Lad explains that disease-process is caused by *doṣas* imbalanced by factors such as unsuitable diet, or smoking, which weaken tissues in specific locations of the body where disease may then take hold. Treatment does not focus on eradication of external pathogenic factors, but rather on restoring the balance of conditions and forces within the affected tissues and system, the system surrounding it, and the whole organism.[21] Āyurveda's theory of pathogenesis implies that a determinant of health is equilibrium of the functions that support undamaged tissues and systems, in order to avoid tendencies to malfunction when pathogens are inevitably encountered.

Contemporary scientific medicine makes particular use of chemical analysis, and here the concept of equilibrium concerns the balance of chemical substances and processes within an organism. Physiological functions depend on chemical factors and interactions whose equilibrium can be evaluated quantitatively. Chemical levels in the body can be analyzed by laboratory procedures and judged in terms of a standard range, with readings falling outside the normal range indicative of particular disorders (e.g., abnormal blood glucose levels may indicate hypoglycemia or diabetes). The pharmaceutical treatment of illness entails introduction of chemical agents into the body to improve functioning and relieve discomfort. Equilibrium in a pharmacological context does not generally entail direct replacement of a particular chemical compound that the body lacks (though in some cases this is so). Rather, the restoration of equilibrium by pharmacology consists in chemically establishing conditions that support normal functions of the body, so that they prevail over factors causing malfunction. Āyurvedic pharmacology emphasizes the patient's particular circumstances in administration of medicines:

> It is necessary to take into account the place where the drugs are produced, the physical conditions of the patient, the appropriate dose of the drug, and the seasonal variation as well as the age of the patient.
>
> AD 1:1.62–63

Āyurvedic diagnosis and treatment invoke the idea of balance not merely for pharmaceutical applications, but as it pertains to the relationship between persons and their environment and life-circumstances. Dash and Junius note that the idea of balance can apply to relationships with family, friends, work, culture, and God.[22] An important application of the idea of equilibrium in the context of health is avoidance of extremes in diet, sleep, work, recreation and other activities.

Adaptation

Medical theorist Claude Bernard, working in the nineteenth-century climate of Lamarck's and Darwin's evolutionary theories, regarded disease as a result of an organism's failure to adapt to environmental insults.[23] Brody and Sobel's *systems-theory of health* assumes Dubos' position that "states of health or disease are the expression of the success or failure experienced by an organism in its effort to respond adaptively to environmental challenges."[24] The systems-theory view of health incorporates various 'levels' or domains, through which information flows in a pattern of feedback loops: "component A influences component B and the new state of B then 'feeds back' to influence A."[25] Brody and Sobel summarize the concept of health as "the ability of a system (e.g., cell, organism, family, society) to respond adaptively to a wide variety of environmental challenges (e.g., physical, chemical, infectious, psychological, social)."[26]

Adaptation in the Darwinian sense of reproductive success is one meaning of adaptation, but adaptation further refers to an organism's having a relation to its environment that is both self-preserving and accomodating of impinging forces. Jozsef Kovács characterizes a healthy relationship between organism and environment as "a dynamic steady state which can be maintained by the living being in spite of changes in the environment."[27] In biological terms, health coincides with the highest stability and self-preservation of the individual and of the species, which in turn contributes to the self-preservation of the ecosystem in which individuals and species participate. In human life, adaptation is not only a biological process; it is also cultural process, involving the production and use of knowledge, instruments, methods, and institutions aimed at successful participation in the environment, and transformation of it.[28]

Adaptation for the purpose of self-preservation is central to Descartes' physics, medicine, and ethics. Descartes' physics is concerned with "simple bodies," what contemporary science calls "masses in motion," and the natural forces that resolve compound bodies back into their original state as simple bodies. In the physical universe, each entity, living or non-living, acts and reacts to its environment so as to maximize its chances of survival. The living organism, in Descartes' terms, is a compound body formed of organ systems, a mechanism of self-preservation that supports the functioning and interaction of those organs. Life, then, is the compound motion of the simple bodies constituting the organism, and medicine is responsible for helping human beings preserve the functions of the body's systems. For Descartes, just as medicine is concerned with relations among the parts of the body, ethics addresses the relations among persons (i.e., living, sentient, compound bodies) so that each might act as an organic part of the largest body, society, or the 'body politic.'[29]

In psychological terms, adaptation pertains to how a person responds to life's problems, classified by Maslow and Mittelmann as (1) biological and physical, (2) cultural, and (3) those set by internal psychological demands.[30] An ambiguity in human health exists in the fact that even though adaptation is generally a criterion of health, there are cases where *failure* to adapt is indicative of health. Sanford gives this example:

> People who adapted to Hitler's Germany of the 1930's appeared "well"; in terms of their particular social framework they were well-adjusted people. Those who could *not* adapt found themselves in a painful condition, and suffered a terrible malaise. They appeared sick and disturbed people, but their very lack of adaptation may well have been their sign of health. It is as though there was too much health in them to adapt to a sick situation.[31]

Medically, disease itself may be adaptive, as in the case of cowpox infection preventing smallpox.[32]

Āyurveda demonstrates that the medical use of the concept of adaptation has been operative from ancient times. Zimmermann translates from *Caraka-saṃhitā* 1:6.50:

> Experts in appropriateness try to oppose a regimen of diet and exercise (literally a *sātmya*) with contrary qualities to those of the places and diseases in question.[33]

Sātmya (*sa* , 'with'; *ātma*, 'self') is translated by Zimmermann as "habituation," and by Sharma and Dash as "homologation" [CS 3:8.118]. 'Homologation' connotes 'making similar' [Gk. *homo-logos*, 'agreeing']. P. V. Sharma translates *oka-sātmya* as "suitability by practice" [CS 3:8.118], and translates its definition as "adjustment to a particular diet or behavior due to practice" [CS 1:6:50]. Zimmermann clarifies: *sātmya* concerns "what has become beneficial to a person through constant use." While biogeographical habituation or *sāmtya* is recommended in a short-term view of the influence of climate, Zimmermann says that "in the long term, however, the practitioner seeks to obtain an immunity through habituation."[34] This second sense of *sātmya* "denotes an intervention made on the patient's body; it has the different meaning of a regimen or remedy which 'compensates' for some excess or lack: a person wasting away is fed on sweet food for example." Based on the Āyurvedic notion of body and land as the two kinds of place (*deśa*), Zimmermann uncovers two dimensions of health-promoting adaptation: *compensation* using contraries in *therapeutic deśasātmya* (applying particular remedies), and *habituation* to external conditions in *biogeographical deśasātmya* (concerning the dietary practices of peoples in different environments).[35] Zimmermann communicates the ethos of Āyurveda in this remark about the adaptation procedure called *sātmya*: "The ideal is to accustom oneself to hit on the right choice of regimen, learned doses, and mixture, so that the nature of what is eaten is rendered appropriate to the nature of the one who eats it."[36]

Non-susceptibility

Biologically, non-susceptibility means resistance or immunity to potentially infectious agents or damaging forces. The *Āyurveda Dīpikā* gives a succinct definition of resistance:

> Resistance to diseases or immunity from diseases includes both attenuation of the manifested diseases as well as prevention of the unmanifested ones.
>
> AD 1:28.7

Non-susceptibility is a determinant of health in that an organism's resistance to infectious or other threatening agents signals its power of persisting in its own functions, while resisting or overcoming the effects of, for example, microorganisms to which it is exposed. Non-susceptibility is also the principle behind participation without injury in activities requiring exertion. Vitality is at the root of resistance to both biological illness and physical injury. Vitality connotes the strength and energy to prevail in one's own being and activities, and withstanding interference from forces in one's environment.

Psychologically, non-susceptibility means a state of mental clarity and equilibrium from which one can respond to pressures from other persons' behaviors and communications, and from within one's own psyche, without extreme reactions of suffering or behavior damaging to self or others. While *vāta*, *pitta*, and *kapha* are pathogenic factors of the body, Āyurveda names two of the three *guṇas* (principles of matter) as the pathogenic factors affecting the mind: *rajas* (activity) and *tamas* (inertia). The *Caraka-saṃhitā* claims as its province physical medicine (not psychological medicine), but nevertheless it recommends "spiritual and scriptural knowledge, patience, memory, and meditation" for reducing susceptibility to maladaptive mental influences [CS 1:1.58].

Vitality, Endurance, and Relaxation

In Āyurveda, the life force is considered to consist in a physiological fluid material called *ojas:*

> It is the *ojas* which keeps all living beings refreshed. There can be no life without *ojas*. It marks the beginning of the formation of the embryo. . . . Loss of *ojas* amounts to loss of life itself. It sustains the life and is located in the heart. It constitutes the essence of all tissue elements. The *elan vital* ['life force'] owes its existence to it.
>
> CS 1:30.9–11

Although Āyurveda understands *ojas* as a physical substance, the word *ojas* also expresses the abstractions we call 'energy' or 'vitality' in human life. Sharma and Dash translate *ojas* as *energy* in this passage of the *Caraka-saṃhitā:* "A body possessed of organs having proper measurement is endowed with longevity, strength, energy (*ojas*), happiness, power, wealth and virtues" [CS 3:8.117]. P. V. Sharma translates *ojas* in this passage as 'immunity.' As a physical substance, *ojas* is the essence of the seven tissue elements: chyle, blood, flesh, fat, bone, marrow, and semen or ova.

> The excellent essence of the *dhātus* beginning with *rasa* (chyle) and ending with semen (*śukra*) or ova and blood (*śoṇita*) is called *ojas*. This *ojas* is also called *bala* (strength) in the context of the medical science. Because of strength, there is stability and nourishment of the muscle tissues and the person remains undeterred in all efforts.[37]

Vitality, from the Latin noun *vita*, life, refers to the force of life. Vitality connotes vigor and strength, and as a determinant of health it represents an entity's strength to assert itself for survival, for meeting challenges and accomplishing chosen purposes. Strength refers to the power of resisting or generating an effect or force. It is an important factor in diagnosis, for loss of strength is often indicative of compromised functioning, though individuals possess and utilize strength in different ways. Endurance is the power to act in a sustained way when a continued expenditure of effort and concentration is required.

Relaxation and stress are significant factors for health, and the concept of vitality provides an interpretive context for them. Tension and relaxation are complementary poles in maintaining homeostasis. In instances ranging over cellular integrity, arterial pressure, and the person's affective sense of sufficient challenge and rest, vitality requires some degree of tension to stimulate action, and to maintain or strengthen an organism's capacities. At the same time, relaxation is imperative for preventing more extreme forms of tension that can damage tissues, systems, and psychological resiliency. Relaxation is not only a means of maintaining vitality, but a sign that an organism is maintaining its functional equilibrium and well-being.

Medical and Psychological Determinants

Normality

In contemporary scientific medicine, a widely applied criterion of health is the 'normal' functioning of an organ, system, or person, with normality established by comparison with bio-statistical data, as articulated in Boorse's theory of health.[38] Normality can be understood in terms of:

1. PATHOLOGY: Normality is defined in terms of presence and extent of disease.
2. STATISTICS: Normality is defined in terms of deviation from the distribution of a given characteristic in a population.
3. SOCIAL VALUES: Normality is determined in relation to values (e.g., the question of whether homosexuality is normal).[39]

The *Caraka-saṃhitā* lists the following determinants of normality as criteria for determining whether a cure has been effected:

- Alleviation of pain
- Normal voice
- Normal complexion
- Increased strength
- Appetite
- Proper digestion, and nourishment of the body
- Proper elimination of waste
- Proper sexual functioning
- Sufficient sleep at the proper time
- Absence of dreams indicating morbidity, happy awakening
- Unimpaired mind, intellect, and sense faculties [CS 3:8.89]

Central to Āyurvedic diagnosis and therapy is restoration of conditions regarded as normal for all persons, but achieved on the basis of what is normal for an individual's particular type of constitution. Because an individual's normal structure and function depend on the equilibrium of the three *doṣas*, what is normal for a given person depends on his or her type of constitution, whether dominated by *vāta* ('wind': the force of motion), *pitta* ('bile': the force of heat), or *kapha* ('phlegm': the force of stability) or a combination of two of these, or all three.

> The entire body is in fact the abode of all the *doṣas* and as such these *doṣas* bring about good and bad results according as they are in normal and abnormal states respectively. When in a normal state, they bring about good results like growth, strength, complexion, happiness, etc. When in an abnormal state they cause various types of diseases.
>
> CS 1:20.9

Health and disease in Āyurveda are relative to the normal and abnormal states of the *doṣas*, and hence the absence or alleviation of disease is coextensive with equilibrium of the *doṣas* suitable to a given person's constitution. The names of the three *doṣas* should not be taken in literal terms as the substances phlegm, bile, and wind, but understood to represent qualities of physiological structures and functions. The three forces governing biological processes in the normal state of equilibrium that constitutes health are traditionally called *dhātus*, 'supports' (√*dhā*, 'to give,' e.g., to give support). Disturbance of the *dhātus'* equilibrium is coextensive with states of compromised health. In disequilibrium the three are called *doṣas* or 'faults' (√ *duṣ*, 'to soil,' 'to spoil,' 'to impair').

> There are two aspects of the *doṣas*, viz., natural and morbid. In the natural state, *pitta* helps in living beings' digestion and metabolism. In its morbid state, it causes various diseases. *Kapha* in its natural state promotes strength in the form of *ojas*. When in morbid condition, it takes the form of excreta and causes misery. Similarly, *vāta* in its natural state is responsible for all activities of the body. When in morbid state, it causes diseases and death.
>
> CS 1:17.115-18

Pharmacist and Āyurvedic researcher Birgit Heyn makes the nontraditional, but clinically useful distinction that the term *dhātu* is properly employed to mean 'tissue-element,' while *doṣa* refers to the dynamic bioenergetic principles: "three different forms of energy which govern the whole energy economy in living organisms."[40] As regards *vāta*, *pitta*, and *kapha* as psychophysical 'types,' these are stylized pictures used as a general guide in recognizing the characteristics of each person's nature, wherein a particular *doṣa* generally predominates.[41]

Zimmermann maintains that in ancient Hindu medicine, the humors were conceived within two superimposed standpoints: First, according to an agricultural metaphor, as fluids irrigating the tissues. Second, in terms of health and disease, they represent various facets in a combinative system of humors, savors, and qualities possessed by humans, animals, plants, and by the soils that infuse plants and animals with their *rasa* ('juice' or essence) throughout the food chain.[42] Thus the ancient Āyurvedic practitioner did not consider the three humors wind, bile, and phlegm in a literal sense, but made a leap of abstraction from the level of image to the construction of a conceptual system. This is "the moment when phlegm is no longer simply an image of excessive serosity or unctuosity, but becomes the abstract principle of elephantiasis."[43]

The several meanings of *doṣa* indicate that understanding and applying Āyurvedic principles requires multileveled analysis. An important clinical interpretation of *doṣa* is excess material resulting from the incomplete digestion of food. The verbal root *duṣ* gives the word *doṣa* the connotation of 'spoiling' or 'impairment.' The stomach, and particularly the gastric 'fire,' may be 'spoiled' owing to faulty digestion. This results in the spreading throughout the body of a sticky substance called *āma*, 'unripe' or incompletely digested food-juice. The *sāma* ('with *āma*') state of the body is marked by the symptoms of "a feeling of heaviness in the body, sleeplessness, sticky stools and saliva, swelling in the body, aches and pains, etc."[44] Daniel C. Tabor reports the explanation of a *vaidya* or Āyurvedic physician who asserts that chronic disorders (e.g., backache) result from *āma* in the body. Acute illnesses (e.g., cholera) have other immediate causes, but proximally, "the predisposition of the body to these infections was held to be caused by *āma* also."[45]

Nirāma (without *āma*) is the state of normality and hence of health. It is indicated by signs including lightness of limb, and proper appetite and elimination. Āyurvedic treatment employs measures to return the body to the normal *nirāma* state before the administration of medicines appropriate for particular disorders. A major therapeutic strategy in Āyurveda is *śamana* or alleviation therapy: elimination of *āma* by rekindling the digestive fire or *agni* (in modern terms: digestive enzymes and processes, along with metabolism). Alleviation therapy includes fasting or light diet, exercise, the drinking of warm water, and adminstration of digestive herbs, singly or in compounds—for instance, dried ginger (*Zingiber officianale*).[46] These procedures reactivate the reciprocally related functions of the gastric fire and elimination, and the 'drying up' of excess *doṣas*.

While normality has many applications as a diagnostic criterion in Āyurvedic and Western medicine, Nietzsche provides another perspective on medical normality. Nietzsche rejects the idea of 'normal health' in general terms. He valued sickness and other morbid states for showing us "under a magnifying glass states that are normal but not easily visible when normal."[47] But as for a standard of 'normal health' Nietzsche says the concept should be abandoned, for what constitutes health for the *body* (let alone the soul) "depends on your goal, your horizon, your energies, your impulses, your errors, and above all on the ideals and phantasms of your soul."[48] With the forsaking of the idea of a normal health, he says, we may reflect on the health and illness of the soul. The sick soul is really necessary, Nietzsche holds, to provoke the growth of our knowledge, self-knowledge, and virtue. Difficulties and suffering can demand our self-reflection and the exercise of our power. An ambiguity thus emerges in the suggestion that while medical science—contemporary or Āyurvedic—relies on a concept of normality as a criterion of health, our 'abnormality' can be a generative factor for healing.

Freedom from Pain

Freedom from pain is a foremost determinant of health, and relieving pain is among the primary goals of medicine. Pain is generally the most prominent and immediate indicator of the presence of illness and injury.

Āyurveda classifies diseases as *exogenous* (caused by external factors, such as fire), and *endogenous* (caused by impairment of the *doṣas*). There are four major subgroups of disease, because exogenous and endogenous diseases may manifest in mind or body [CS 1:20.3]. As regards pain:

> The exogenous diseases begin with pain, and then they bring about disturbance in the equilibrium of the *doṣas*. The endogenous diseases on the other hand, begin with disturbance in the equilibrium of *doṣas* and then bring about pain.
>
> CS 1:20.7

Pain more often than not accompanies illness and injury; we associate pain with disease, and freedom from pain with health. However, pain and disease are not coextensive: Pain may occur to persons in good health, and illness may be present without accompanying pain or immediate suffering, for example, in the case of hypertension. Drew Leder's phenomenological analysis of the body and its "dys-appearance" in its ordinary states of well-being reveals the experienced dimensions of pain and disease:

> The body stands out in times of dysfunction only because its usual state is to be lost in the world—caught up in a web of organic and intentional involvements through which we form one body with other things. To say that the body is "absent," a "being-away," thus has a positive significance; it asserts that the body is in ceaseless relation to the world.[49]

Our associating pain with disease, Leder says, is not due merely to their occurring together in time. A phenomenological association occurs as well. "Disease tends to effect many of the same experiential shifts as does pain"; disease and pain bring about disruption of our intentional links with the world, and can constrict our spatiotemporal horizons.[50]

An ambiguity regarding pain exists in the fact that pain, while generally undesirable, is critical to health, for it signals the presence of threats to health.[51] Another ambiguity pertinent to pain is the fact that pain often goes unrecognized. This claim might seem surprising, for the meaning of 'pain' connotes the characteristic of being *felt*. However, it commonly occurs that persons experience pain without accompanying awareness of its existence, location, and severity. Diminished or delayed awareness of pain can be a sign of a low degree of body awareness, sometimes caused by a high degree of involvement in one's mental processes. (However, the ability to mentally control pain can be an aspect of healthiness.) In either case, *awareness*, discussed subsequently, presents itself as a determinant of health: awareness is both a determinant of health and a resource for protecting and improving one's health.

In psychological terms, physical pain and mental suffering can be results of a person's subjection to injurious forces outside his or her control—another's abusive behavior, for example—or they can arise from tensions in a person's own psyche. As Nietzsche says, however, psychological suffering can have the productive quality of provoking a person's development.

The motive to avoid pain (physical and/or psychological) can lead to reliance on alcohol or drugs, prescribed or non-prescribed. Physical debilitation is a possible consequence of substance abuse, and other kinds of damage can result from abusing drugs. Spiritually, substance abuse can cloud a person's motivation and clarity of understanding. Morally, it can interfere with the making and fulfilling of commitments. Alleviation of suffering without reflection on its meaning neglects its positive value to provide information about physical health problems. Additionally, it can involve overlooking the potential of psychological suffering to incite the development of personhood and maturity.

Wholeness and Integration

Āyurveda's medical holism is founded on a cosmology wherein the person is a microcosm of the macrocosmic world, a position that has religious as well as medical implications:

> An individual is an epitome of the universe, as all the material and spiritual phenomena of the universe are present in the individual, and all those present in the individual are also contained in the universe. . . . As soon as he realizes his identity with the entire universe, he is in possession of true knowledge which stands him in good stead in getting salvation.
>
> CS 4:5.3, 7

Āyurveda considers the universe (and all matter in it, including human beings) to be compounded of the basic substances earth, water, fire, air, and *ākāśa* ('ether' or space), and *Brahman* or supreme consciousness [CS 4:5.3–5]. On this metaphysical basis, Āyurvedic therapeutics aim to restore the *doṣas*' equilibrium in consideration of influences such as season, climate, and local foodstuffs and medicinal substances. Classical Āyurvedic pharmacology recommends medicinal substances conditioned by the environment, and holds that the *rasa* or essence of foods and medicines (gained from the *rasa* of the soil in which they grew) pervades the *rasa* or essence that is the basis of the human's seven *dhātus* or tissues.[52]

The word 'health' actually means wholeness, and 'to heal' is to restore wholeness. *Health*, *heal*, and *whole* are derived from the Old English *hāl*, 'whole,' and ultimately descend from the Indo-European root meaning whole: √ *kailo-*.[53] Holism is a conceptual orientation that recognizes the organic unity and interdependence of forces within an organism, among organisms, and among forces at various levels within an environment.

> . . . a holistic approach offers a conceptual alternative to the physiochemical reductionism, materialism, and mind/body dualism that dominates much of contemporary medical thought.[54]

Besides its ontological dimension, holism also pertains to function. Leon R. Kass connects wholeness with *well-working:* wholeness as regards living organisms is not static, but pertains to wholeness-in-action, the working well of the entity; thus the whole organism must be evaluated in order to determine its well-working.[55] Kass' interpretation of wholeness is more satisfactory than interpretations that define wholeness statically. By regarding wholeness from the standpoint of well-working, the concept of wholeness becomes more useful as a criterion of health. For instance, a person who lacks the ability to hear can still attain to wholeness by virtue of using means of communication that enable her to carry out projects of importance to her.

In the psychological theory of Carl G. Jung, the journey toward wholeness, which he called individuation, is a process involving the bringing to consciousness of meanings previously repressed in the unconscious. Psychological health in Jungian terms entails that one's inner and outer selves are integrated rather than fragmented.

> As long as all goes well and psychic energy finds its application in adequate and well-regulated ways, we are disturbed by nothing from within. . . . But no sooner are one or two of the channels of psychic activity blocked, than we are reminded of a stream that is dammed up. The current flows backward to its source; the inner man wants something which the visible man does not want, and we are at war with ourselves.[56]

Wholeness describes an ideal state, for life circumstances change constantly and require new adjustments and responses. Further, our human potential can never be fully achieved in our lifetimes and, in this respect, achieving wholeness is impossible, because the possibilities for our development are so rich.[57] Wholeness, then, like the concept of health itself, is a conceptual rubric and regulative idea, that is—an action-guiding ideal. Wholeness is a significant determinant of health, for it sets a standard for judging the extent to which a person is fully acting and experiencing.

One way of understanding *integration* is in terms of the concept of wholeness: To integrate is to make something whole by bringing its parts into proper relation. The Latin adjective *integer* (from the Indo-European root √ *tag*, 'to touch') means 'untouched,' hence, whole, complete, and perfect.[58] *Integer* is the basis of the English nouns *integer* (whole number), and *integrity* (moral consistency and soundness). Āyurveda suggests that integration is fundamental to health by its use of the term *roga* for illness. *Roga* is derived from the verbal root √ *ruj*, 'to break,' while its negated form, *ārogya*, means health. Integration, like wholeness, is more fruitfully considered in dynamic rather than static terms. As a determinant of health, integration pertains to the degree of cooperation within and among the systems, subsystems, and constituent parts of an entity.

Loss of integration characterizes illness and injury in that the affected part stands out in its dysfunction. Leder refers to this phenomenon as a *thematization:* pain brings the body out of its well-working 'absent' state to an experience of intense awareness of the affected part. Leder invokes Heidegger's reference to the "ready-to-hand" tool (*Being and Time*, 95–107). The tool remains withdrawn from our attention as long as it serves the purpose of our work, the "towards-which" the tool is used. In the same way that a tool stands forth due to a break in its usefulness, "it is characteristic of the body itself to presence in times of breakdown or problematic performance."[59] Leder gives the example of a person who has a heart attack while playing tennis:

> Prior to the onset of pain . . . attention is ecstatically distributed to the distant points. Parts of the body are backgrounded and forgotten as all power centers in the swing. A metabolic machinery supplies the player with energy, without demanding his attention or guidance. The game is made possible only by this bodily self-concealment. Yet this structure is lacerated by a single moment of pain. The player is called back from ecstatic engagement to a focus upon the state of his own body. A background region, the chest, is now thematized.[60]

Leder uses the terms *disappearance* and *dys-appearance* to characterize the body in its states of well-working and dysfunction, respectively. He capitalizes on the etymological difference between the Latin prefix *dis*, meaning 'away,' 'apart,' or 'asunder,' and the Greek prefix *dys*, meaning 'bad,' 'difficult,' or 'ill,' as in 'dysentery.' Disappearance evokes absence, and refers to the state of ordinary functioning where the lived-body is 'absent' from awareness due to its ecstatic involvement in its projects in the world. In contrast, 'dys-appearance' refers to states where "the body *appears* as thematic focus, but precisely in a *dys* state."[61]

Integration characterizes the state of health and well-working, while dys-appearance, the thematized appearance of an impaired part or system of the body, is equivalent to dis-integration in the function of the body as whole. Hegel's definition of the disease-state turns on such an idea of integration:

> . . . the system or organ establishes itself in isolation, and by persisting in its particular activity in opposition to the activity of the whole, obstructs the activity, as well as the process by which it pervades all the moments of the whole.[62]

In considering integration as a determinant of health, it seems at first a simple matter that integration is a mark of health, and disintegration a mark of illness. But Leder's analysis reveals that both illness and health involve a certain kind of disintegration that takes the form of alienation from one's own body:

> Both exhibit an element of alienation from the body. In the case of health, the body is alien by virtue of its disappearance, as attention is primarily directed toward the world. With the onset of illness this gives way to dys-appearance. The body is no longer alien-as-forgotten, but precisely as-remembered, a sharp and searing presence threatening the self. One is a mode of silence, the other a manner of speech, yet they are complementary and correlative phenomena.[63]

Leder's insight is useful to understanding yet another of the ambiguities inherent in the experience of human health and illness: health can permit a degree of integration with our projects (whether in the world or in the spiritual domain) that diminishes the integration of body with consciousness. For instance, classical Yoga cultivates health as a condition for meditative practice aimed at *dis-integration* of bonds keeping the consciousness connected with body and senses.

Awareness and Mental Clarity

Awareness in the context of health has a number of applications. A healthy organism has capacities for sensory awareness, while illness or injury can interfere with the organism's ability to register information in its environment. An extreme example is loss of consciousness due to injury or illness, and gradual loss of awareness is one of the signs of impending death. *The Bṛhadāraṇyaka Upaniṣad* describes the soul at death as becoming "non-knowing of forms." "He is becoming one," they say, "he does not see . . . (smell, etc.)" [Bṛhad. Up. 4:4.1–2]. The *Chāndogya*

Upaniṣad [6:15.1] describes how the relatives of a dying person gather and ask "Do you know me?" For in the final phases of dying, it commonly occurs that dying persons lose awareness sufficient even to recognize their loved ones.

Among the criteria for evaluating whether a cure has been effected, the *Caraka-saṃhitā* lists "unimpairment of mind, intellect, and senses" [CS 3:8.89]. The Hindu traditions, in various terms, uphold the position that intelligence or consciousness is the person's true nature, and that discriminative wisdom is the remedy for the ignorance, suffering, and bondage that is human life. Thus it is not surprising that Āyurveda considers the pain of illness to result from ignorance, and holds that clarity of mind is a determinant of health. Clarity of mind in the context of health is an ordinary kind of knowledge, not a form of higher knowledge leading to religious liberation; mental clarity contributes to liberation from the suffering of illness:

> . . . the ignorant indulge in unwholesome gratification of the five senses . . . and adoption of such regimens as are pleasing only temporarily; but the wise do not indulge in them because of their clarity of vision.
>
> CS 1:28.39–40

Awareness is a determinant of health, and a capacity that contributes to the maintenance of health: Āyurvedic medical theory implies that knowledge of one's own nature, and the dietary, climatic, temporal, and other patterns suited to oneself helps a person follow the proper regimen to preserve health. The *Caraka-saṃhitā* gives this analogy to illustrate the principles of self-awareness and responsibility for one's state of health: "As an incompetent king neglects his enemy, so also an ignorant person does not realize the need to take care of the disease in its primary stage due to his negligence" [CS 1:11.57]. Awareness of one's normal functioning and deviations from it can help one sustain a higher level of health, and to recognize circumstances that signal a need for adjustment in one's actions or a need for medical assistance.

In the domain of psychological health, awareness and clarity of mind are contrary to neurosis and psychosis. Psychological disorders involve internal conflicts far from transparent to their sufferer, and psychosis is marked by interference in a person's contact with reality. An important dimension of mental health is a person's awareness of his or her own thoughts and feelings, and a certain degree of awareness (free of projection and other neurotic interpretations) of others' emotions and communications. Psychological health entails mental clarity sufficient for responding appropriately to experiences and communications. In contrast, neurotic behavior is often impelled by interpretations fueled by unconscious inner tensions, and thus can be inappropriate to a given situation. Inner psychological tensions spring from, and produce, suffering. Neurotic or psychotic behaviors tend to produce further suffering in both the subject and those with whom he or she interacts. The Hindu postulate that suffering is rooted in ignorance is supported by the efficacy of psychotherapy to relieve psychological suffering through replacing nescience of one's own psyche with self-understanding.

In addition to the direct applications of awareness for attainment and preservation of health, awareness in contradistinction to self-deception is an aspect of having a healthy connection with truth in the achievement of personhood. Deutsch articulates self-deception as follows:

> Self-deception is a refusal to acknowledge who I am and what I am doing, not out of simple ignorance but from what appears to be a kind of unselfconscious willful perversity.[64]

Deutsch develops Fingarette's view of self-deception, "that the deceiver is one who refuses to spell out, to avow, some feature of his engagement with the world."[65]

Deutsch distinguishes a number of forms of self-deception, which in its primary forms involves

> . . . breakdown of an individual's capacity to be responsible, to be able (and not just unwilling) to acknowledge the actualities of his or her personal identity making and to exercise one's inherent powers to strive toward integration and freedom.[66]

If we conceive health broadly as well-being encompassing the achievement of personhood, Deutsch's thought on self-deception shows how well-being is countered by self-fragmentation. Self-deception as a form of metaphysical illness finds intelligibility within an understanding of health whose determinants include integration.

Finally, the ability to learn has its genesis in awareness. An organism's health is reflected in, and protected by, its ability (appropriate to its species and situation) to interpret and remember experiences, for purposes ranging from survival, to application of high levels of insight, creativity, and problem-solving. Because of the human being's potential for higher order thinking, aesthetic experience, and so on, the ideal of a high degree of health entails development of the mind's capacities and the exercise of creative potential. The ideal of cultural health thus requires that societies have effective schools for the cultivation of human intelligence and its applications, especially for the young, but ideally for lifelong learning.

Sociocultural and Aesthetic Determinants

Relationality

Relationality signifies relationships of various kinds: interpersonal, between person and society, among social groups and nations, and between persons and other kinds of beings (living and non-living) who constitute the world. Psychology and sociology investigate relations among persons and groups, social and political theorists discuss relationality in the sociopolitical domain, and ethicists in terms of morality. But relationality can be understood in some other and interestingly subtle ways.

Self-sufficiency is a determinant of health, and in evaluating a person's health, an important question is: How much does a given condition interfere with the person's ability to act independently to accomplish his or her purposes? A limited capacity to act can indicate a compromised state of health. On the other hand, health as a positive state is relative to the power to act in one's own behalf to meet one's needs and desires. Moreover, because our humanity entails the duties and benefits of community life, vitality can be employed in one's work and social service to contribute to the well-being of others. Self-sufficiency is important to health, but its necessary condition is relationality, a concept that illuminates meanings of health as regards person, species, environment, and community.

The notion of 'social determinants of health' suggests two main themes; the first is social factors as they bear on medical health. It was in this connection that Descartes envisaged a social revolution based on medicine, consonant with Rudolph Virchow's concept of the role of health in democratic government:

> The democratic state desires that all its citizens enjoy a state of well-being, for it recognizes that they all have equal rights. . . . However, the conditions of well-being are health and education, so it is the task of the state to provide on the broadest possible basis the means for maintaining and promoting health and education through public action.[67]

The second theme emergent in the idea of social determinants of health is the one emphasized here: perspectives on what it means to be healthy in context of human social and cultural life—that is, creation of meanings based on values concerning relationality and aesthetics. For varied insights into relationality, we may turn to sources including Āyurveda, Neo-Confucianism, and indigenous religious cosmologies. Leder's study of medical and philosophical dimensions of the body utilizes Neo-Confucianism as a tradition grounded in relationality, and draws on Wang Yang-ming's description of the universal empathy whereby we may "form one body" with all things:

> Everything from ruler, minister, husband, wife, and friends to mountains, rivers, spiritual beings, birds, animals, and plants should be truly loved in order to realize my humanity that forms one body with them, and then my clear character will be completely manifested, and I will really form one body with Heaven, Earth, and the myriad things.[68]

Leder invokes against the Cartesian mechanistic model of the body, the Neo-Confucian principle of relationality. He recommends three ways whereby we may "form one body": morally, by *compassion*, aesthetically, by *absorption* or aesthetic openness to the world, and spiritually, by *communion*, experiencing "interconnection with the ground of all being."[69]

Descartes' medical philosophy is mechanistic, yet at the same time organic—in other words, relational. The human body as the subject of medical science he conceived in terms of a machine, governed by the principles of physics, and subject to physical manipulations to restore it to proper functioning. However, Descartes has an organic view of the inter-relation of the organs and systems of the individual body, and the inter-relation of persons who together constitute the body of society. Health in Descartes' view depends on the concern of the mind to conserve the union of body and soul. According to Cartesian physics, God created the world, and it continues to exist because God continually "conserves" it.[70] The human body is fit to receive a soul by virtue of the interconnection of its organ systems; the conservation of the union of soul and body is afforded by the mind's concern for the preservation of life, and by supportive factors in the environment.[71] Along similar lines, Descartes holds that political association is an instrument for the conservation of its human constituents. Its institutions can be regarded as organs of the body politic, and the body politic serves in turn to preserve the soul-body unions of the persons who constitute it.[72] In addition to relationality's inclusion of ethical relations among persons, a vast topic not undertaken here, relationality characterizes cosmologies envisaging an interconnected web of life.

Āyurveda illuminates the idea of relationality as a determinant of health. Gerald Larson identifies several possibilities for expanding our concepts of the self and the human species, and our valuation of the ecology of the living world. In suggesting new agendas for healing based on Āyurvedic and South Asian cultural axioms, Larson employs the logical concept of *abhāva*, 'analytic absence' to suggest the following perspectives on person, species, and life:

Axiom 1 Absence of separation between birth and rebirth

The person is a product not just of parents, and of action in the present life, but of karmic heritage stemming from former lives, perhaps expressible in modern terms of evolutionary trajectory.

In terms of relationality, an 'individual' exists in relation to past and future instantiations of her/himself.

Axiom 2 Absence of separation between self and self, or self and other

Hindu concepts including ādhibhautika *(sociality) could inform a socio-biological notion of 'species-health.'*

Relationality functions in the capacity of pointing out transactional and 'dividual' influences on human health.

Axiom 3 Absence of separation between divine and human, or between one species and another

The idea of rebirth in another life-form could ground "an ecological reverence for life that encompasses more than the human."[73]

Applications of relationality within ecologically grounded conceptions of life and health are precisely what is needed in our present world to address the compromised and threatened well-being of ecosystems and their inhabitants.

Relationality is a motif in both contemporary ecological theory and philosophy of health. In ancient times, Āyurveda used ideas of relationality in an ecologically informed approach to medicine. Ancient Hindu ecology conceived the land and the human body as the two kinds of place. Ecology was integral to the practice of a pathology based not on scientific physiology (which 2000 years ago had not yet evolved in India nor Greece), but on *prognosis*, the interpretation of symptoms and stages of an illness. Zimmermann writes that the physician proceeded by "taking into consideration the most general conditions of life: climate, seasons, customs, postures. Ecology was an integral part of this practical context."[74]

The volume of the *Caraka-saṃhitā* dealing with the body is the fourth volume, *Śarīra-sthāna* (*śarīra:* body). It has chapters on mind and soul, embryology, anatomy, obstetrics, and pediatrics. In its fifth chapter, *Puruṣavicaya Śarīra*, "Individual and Universe," is this verse that expresses the cosmological and pragmatic significance of relationality:

> If one realizes himself as spread in the entire universe and the entire universe spread in himself, he is indeed in possession of transcendental and worldly vision. His serenity of mind based on wisdom never fades away.
> CS 4:5.20

Creativity

In Chopra's articulation of Āyurveda, life itself is creativity, and healing is a creative act. The body, its systems, and its very cells have creative intelligence. At a quantum level, we are continually creating ourselves, physically and with our intelligence.[75] To illustrate the operation of creativity in human physiology, Chopra cites Claude Bernard, who described how the laws of physics and biochemistry "subordinate themselves and succeed one another in a pattern, and according to a law which pre-exists; they repeat themselves with order, regularity, constancy, and they harmonize in such a manner as to bring about the organization and growth of the individual."[76] Chopra conceives disease as diversion from the flow of intelligence,[77] and he sees creative intelligence as a key to health, that is, to creating conditions for new and more successful patterns in the functioning of the body/mind. In his work on aging and longevity, Chopra connects creativity with the universal force of creation. Invoking the traditional Hindu view of the three forces by which the universe exists—creation, maintenance, and destruction—Chopra writes:

> The genes of every species include the code for creating new cells, maintaining each cell for a certain time, and destroying it to make way for another generation of tissue. This three-in-one intelligence is what you are trying to affect when you consciously shape your life; it is up to you which aspect—creation, maintenance, or destruction—is most dominant. . . . As long as creation dominates your existence, you will keep growing and evolving.[78]

As regards creativity conceived in the usual sense of realizing and expressing new meanings, Chopra recommends creative activity for elders who wish to maximize their vitality, to create themselves as persons manifesting as much as possible their true human nature in intelligence and bliss. If health is conceived as inclusive of the exercise of one's capacities, then health encompasses creativity. Human beings in general have a high degree of intelligence and a vast range of potential, so a healthy person uses these powers in some creative way suited to her nature. The manifestation of creativity can mark a psychophysical state in which requirements for basic functioning are met, and a surplus of energy permits the bringing forth of new connections of meaning, whether in thought, language, music, the plastic arts, political participation, or other ways.

Among the ambiguities of human life revealed by consideration of health and illness is the fact, pointed out by Nietzsche, that pain and suffering can be stimulants to creativity. Walter Kaufmann says of Nietzsche's dialectical conception of health:

> It would be absurd to say that the work of healthy artists is *eo ipso* beautiful, while that of the ill must be ugly. . . . Homer was blind and Beethoven deaf. Even Shakespeare and Goethe—Nietzsche thinks—must have experienced a profound defect: artistic creation is prompted by something which the artist lacks, by suffering rather than undisturbed good health, by "sicknesses as great stimulants to life" (*The Will to Power*, 1003).[79]

In contrast to Nietzsche's view, Deutsch describes creativity in terms of the imparting of vitality:

> The creative act is a kind of "letting be," but at the same time it is a shaping, a formative act, that involves expressive power. Together with immanent purposiveness and cooperative control, the creative act is an infusion of power, an imparting of a felt life or vitality; it is a making of that which is alive with the very nature of natural-spiritual life.[80]

Deutsch's idea of *creative being* pertains to creative transformation of the constraints and conditions of one's being in the articulation and achievement of personhood.[81] Personal identity and freedom, he claims, are contingent on creative being. Identity and freedom are determinants of creative being, and they are determinants of health, in both medical and religious terms, as will be argued in the following chapter.

Generativity

In biological terms, a determinant of health is the ability to produce offspring. The *Caraka-saṃhitā* addresses reproductive generativity in its sixth volume, *Cikitsā-sthāna:* A person without children is compared to "a lamp in sketches" (not the actual lamp that emanates light). But a person with many children is said to have "many faces, many dimensions, and multi-dimensional knowledge" [CS 6:2, quarter-chapter 1:16–24]. Generativity is presented here under the heading of social and cultural determinants of health rather than biological determinants, because human beings have capacities of spirituality, intellect, and creativity extending beyond our mere biological natures.

To generate is to bring into being, but there are ways other than biological reproduction whereby persons may express generativity. This idea is as ancient as Plato's *Symposium*, wherein Diotima instructs Socrates that some persons' procreancy is of the body, while others' is of the soul. These persons "conceive and bear things of the spirit."

> And what are they? you ask. Wisdom and her sister virtues; it is the office of every poet to beget them, and of every artist whom we may call creative. Now, by far the most important kind of wisdom, she went on, is that which governs the ordering of society, and which goes by the names of justice and moderation.[82]

The developmental theory of Erik Erikson provides a modern psychological articulation of generativity, which Erikson says "encompasses the evolutionary development which has man the teaching and instituting as well as the learning animal."

> Mature man needs to be needed, and maturity needs guidance as well as encouragement from what has been produced and must be taken care of. Generativity, then, is primarily the concern in establishing and guiding the next generation, although there are individuals who through misfortune or because of special and genuine gifts in other directions, do not apply this drive to their own offspring. And indeed, the concept of generativity is meant to include such more popular synonyms as *productivity* and *creativity*, which, however, cannot replace it.[83]

Generativity manifests an individual's vitality by exercising his or her inner resources and initiative to take responsibility for the perpetuation of human culture. Whether or not a person has biological offspring, generativity represents one's participation in the bringing up of new generations. In the present state of the planet, overpopulation is at the root of many of our ills, environmental and human. Thus generativity has an amplified significance as an option for augmenting or transforming the impulse toward biological parenthood in ways that contribute to the well-being of the next generation, without necessarily adding to its numbers.

Enjoyment

The *Caraka-saṃhitā's* recapitulation of the nature of the happy life promoted by Āyurveda lists a number of forms of enjoyment, including strength, knowledge, use of sensory capacities and objects of enjoyment, freedom to achieve, and freedom to move as one likes. The first-listed element of a happy life is freedom from physical and mental ailments [CS 1:30.24]. An account of health would lack an essential ingredient of well-being without the factor of enjoyment. Maslow and Mittelmann note that an aspect of a healthy personality is "interest in several activities" and they list among their criteria for psychological health "the ability to derive pleasure from the physical things in life, such as eating and sleeping."[84]

The idea of enjoyment is applicable in contexts beyond basic physical and psychological ones. Domains of healthful enjoyment include, for example, sport and other forms of recreation, appreciation of the beauty of the natural world, the arts, crafting, friendship and social life, love and sensuality. Enjoyment can characterize the experiencing of meaning and well-being derived from one's work, one's contributions to family and society, and one's spiritual practice. To take the perspective of the *Bhagavadgītā's* Karma Yoga, 'enjoyment' in these aspects of life is not a matter of pleasure, but more a sense of satisfaction from carrying out one's responsibilities.

The aesthetic enjoyment advocated for health in the *Caraka-saṃhitā* includes the wearing of clean, attractive clothing: "It brings about pleasure, grace, competence to participate in conferences, and good appearance." Also recommended are the wearing of scents and jewelry for the experience and expression of pleasantness [CS 1:5.95–97].

Metaphysical and Religious Determinants

Self-identity

Self-identity as a determinant of health signifies the existential problem of knowing one's true nature, and manifesting it in one's being. In the context of health, self-identity encompasses questions about the extent to which a person's health-circumstances permit the seeking and actualizing of Self-nature. In Tillich's analysis of the meaning of health, self-identity is integral to the dialectic process of life in physical, psychological, and other dimensions:

> A centered and balanced living whole goes beyond itself, separates itself partly from its unity, but in so doing it tries to preserve its identity and to return in its separated parts to itself.[85]

The dangers of this dialectical process are, on the one hand, extending oneself in such a way that self-identity is reduced or destroyed, and on the other hand, experiencing various degrees of inability to extend and alter oneself. Thus tension exists in facing possible threats to self-identity (and to one's health, physical and/or psychological) in the course of seeking to realize one's identity.

Nietzsche's point that what is healthy depends on a particular person's nature[86] is echoed in Ingmar Pörn's "Equilibrium Model of Health," which presupposes self-identity as a determinant of health. By 'equilibrium' Pörn means the balance of an individual's capacities and goals. To determine the criteria for a person's health, Pörn says, requires choosing among interpretations of "functioning well," for instance, functioning as one's cohorts do, to meet one's basic needs, or to satisfy one's aspirations. Pörn selects the third interpretation, and defines health as follows:

> Health is the state of a person which obtains when his repertoire [of abilities] is adequate relative to his profile of goals. A person who is healthy in this sense carries with him the intrapersonal resources that are sufficient for what his goals require of *him*.[87]

Health, in Pörns's view, depends on the mutual fitness of a person's profile of goals and his repertoire of abilities. Illness, then, is the state where the repertoire is inadequate to the person's goal profile. Impairments, injuries, and diseases are characterized in Pörn's model as *states*, *changes*, and *processes,* respectively, which are abnormal due to their tendencies to restrict repertoires of desired action. On this basis, one is ill only if one's repertoire is restricted relative to one's own goals. Pörn sees health in relation to a person's ability to do the things that the person holds as goals. If goals are taken to represent steps in the evolution of a person's nature, then working toward goals is a means of articulating one's self-identity. To be healthy is to conduct and cultivate oneself in accord with the truth of one's Self-nature.

Identity is the link between medical and religious therapeutics as analyzed by Halbfass. Regarding a verse in the *Caraka-saṃhitā* concerning the fourfold medical paradigm—*cause*, *diagnosis*, *cure*, and *prevention* of disease—[CS 1:9.19], Halbfass observes that the verse:

> . . . does not mention "health" as such; instead it refers to the "nonrecurrence of diseases" (*rogāṇām apunarbhavaḥ*). While this is a negative manner of expression and presentation, it also contains a remarkable absolutist claim. It is obviously reminiscent of the claims and ideas of

> the philosophers, who try to achieve final liberation from all cyclical occurrences from rebirth and repeated existence (*punarjanma*, *punarbhava*), from *saṃsāra* in general.[88]

Exploring the relation of liberation and identity in Advaita Vedānta, Halbfass quotes Śaṅkara's commentator Sureśvara:

> From medical treatment, the natural state (*svāsthya)* results for one who is afflicted by disease; likewise isolation (*kaivalya*, i.e., final liberation) results once the misconception of the self has been destroyed through knowledge.[89]

Deutsch writes that the possibility of freedom is limited to the extent that self-deception interferes with one's achievement of identity as an integrated person. Self-deception "touches almost everyone in fundamental ways and makes for the spiritual atrophy that so often resides in our being."[90] Realization of identity is a corollary of freedom in the contexts of medical and religious well-being, and to a great extent, identity and freedom embody the meaning of health—both psychophysical and spiritual.

Freedom

Freedom in the domain of physical health refers to freedom from impairments resulting from illness or injury, freedom from accompanying pain and suffering, and freedom from susceptibility. Engelhardt identifies freedom as the essence of health, and concludes that treating medical problems is a matter of granting freedom:

> If health is a state of freedom from the compulsion of psychological and physiological forces, there is a common leitmotif in the treatment of either schizophrenia or congestive heart failure—namely the focus on securing the autonomy of the individual from a particular class of restrictions.[91]

Freedom is a determinant of health because it is a condition for a person to act for survival and the achievement of goals. Psychological freedom concerns a person's inner powers, and the constraints emergent from one's personality and circumstances. Aspects of the personality unaccepted by the self, and submerged in the unconscious, can restrict freedom by interfering with creativity, intimacy, and other articulations of personhood. Non-integrated forces may demand a channeling of effort toward repressing and/or maladaptively engaging those aspects of personality in outer experience. Freedom in the context of psychological health is exemplified by Jung's conception of seeking greater wholeness through bringing to the light of consciousness and integrating into one's awareness restricted and restricting forces of the unconscious.

Freedom is an integral concern in embodied human life and for medicine and the healing arts. Āyurveda is concerned with perpetuating freedom—medical, but also spiritual. Cromwell Crawford identifies the following three themes in his analysis of medical and religious elements of Hindu medicine:

1. Spirituality represents a dimension of health (as do the body and the mind).
2. Spirituality . . . is not isolated from the mind-body complex, but embraces and empowers every cell and fiber of the organism.
3. The relationship of spirituality to health is reciprocal—health promotes spirituality and spirituality promotes health.[92]

Concern for freedom is at the heart of Hinduism—freedom from suffering, and from all that interferes with realizing one's true nature. Āyurveda's province is the art and science of medicine; its first priority is not religious liberation, but the immediate issues of health and sickness of the body. Although Āyurveda is not primarily a *mokṣa-śāstra* or science of liberation, liberation is among the Hindu aims of life that Āyurveda seeks to serve, along with material well-being, enjoyment, and righteousness. The *Carara-saṃhitā* refers to the goal of liberation [e.g., CS 4:5.6–7], and advises against skepticism regarding the existence of the other world [1:11.6–33]. However, Āyurveda's immediate focus is freedom in embodied life: freedom from physical and psychological afflictions, and freedom to achieve one's aims. "The happy person . . . has achieved desired results of all actions and moves about where s/he likes" [CS 4:30.24]. One's ultimate aim might be earthly health, wealth, and enjoyment, or it might be spiritual liberation, but either goal is assisted by the wholesome life and strength attainable by application of Āyurvedic principles.

ĀYURVEDIC RELIGIOUS THERAPEUTICS

Fascinating controversies surround the religious and scientific origins and development of Āyurveda. In the words of Kenneth Zysk, Debiprasad Chattopadhyaya rightly argues that

> . . . Indian medical epistemology is fundamentally opposed to brahmanic ideology, and that the classical medical treatises of Caraka and Suśruta result from a grafting process whereby orthodox brahmanic ideals were superimposed onto a medical framework.[93]

Zysk argues that Hindu medicine developed largely by the efforts of heterodox ascetics rather than brahmanic intellectuals, and that Buddhist monastic establishments were highly instrumental in the refinement and systematization of ancient Indian medicine. Reasons for this include the facts that Buddhism is free of injunctions against contact with 'impurity,' and Buddhism's emphasis on compassion and the ethical duty to relieve suffering. While the history of Āyurveda is beyond the scope of this study, our next step here is to consider elements of religious therapeutics in Āyurveda.

Āyurveda is not a *mokṣa-śāstra* or discipline of liberation, but it is a religious therapeutic on three grounds:

1. A tradition of religious philosophy informs its metaphysical and medical concepts.
2. The healing it offers can assist in the quest to achieve ultimate religious liberation.
3. It conceives of wholesome life as itself a kind of holy life.

Āyurveda qualifies as a system of religious therapeutics on the basis that a religious tradition, Hinduism, informs its concepts of person and body as well as its medical theory and practice. Regardless of the exact relationship between Āyurveda's religious and scientific elements, the healthful life promoted by Āyurveda can contribute to spiritual life. Āyurveda presents itself as serving especially the first three of Hinduism's four aims of life. Although its focus on the physical body is an aspect of *artha,* material well-being, the four aims are integral members of a life-plan in which the ultimate goal is *mokṣa* (liberation). The three prior members, *artha* (material well-being), *kāma* (pleasure), and *dharma* (morality), while intrinsically valuable, function also to support the achievement of *mokṣa.* Finally, living according to Āyurvedic principles means living a spiritual life in the sense of achieving a proper relation with what is sacred, and in making *more* of oneself in connection with that sacred force. For Āyurveda, life itself is sacred.

Āyurveda recommends a life that is wholesome, and thus holy, in respect of living according to a pattern of daily and seasonal routines, hygiene, diet, and activities appropriate to one's individual constitution, and nourishing to one's vital energies. At the foundation of such a life is the Hindu principle of self-knowledge. Āyurveda prescribes self-knowledge at an empirical level. The Āyurvedic foundation of self health-care is knowledge: knowledge of the principles of nature that govern health, and knowledge of one's own psychophysical nature and requirements for optimum well-being. Moreover, self-knowledge in Āyurveda functions within a context of religious meaning: the Self that one cares for is a spirit supported by a physical body.

Āyurveda recommends that we adopt ways of living that support our vitality, rather than compromising it. One means of doing this is to regulate one's life in accordance with the qualities of the seasons and times of day. Time is a significant factor in Āyurveda's conception of the causes of disease and health:

> The causes of disease relating to both mind and body are three-fold: wrong utilization, non-utilization and excessive utilization of time, mental faculties, and objects of the sense organs.
>
> The body and mind constitute the substrata of diseases and happiness (i.e., positive health). Balanced utilization (of time, mental faculties and objects of sense organs) is the cause of happiness.
>
> CS 1:54–55

In Āyurvedic self health-care, the factor of time especially concerns attunement with qualities of energy that prevail in particular cycles of the day and year. Information about daily and seasonal regimens is available in the *Caraka-saṃhitā*[94] and other primary sources, but there are good contemporary works on Āyurvedic health maintenance that make Āyurvedic principles more accessible. For an example of the Āyurvedic approach to living in accord with daily time-cycles, and in order to appreciate Āyurvedic principles more concretely, consider some of Chopra's recommendations for daily routine.

Appreciation of Āyurveda's prescription for daily routine requires reference to the three *doṣas* or vital principles, *vāta*, *pitta*, and *kapha*, whose basic natures are motion, metabolism, and stability, respectively. These *doṣas* govern a three-phase cycle between sunrise and sunset, which is repeated during the hours of darkness between sunset and sunrise. By waking before sunrise, "you take advantage of Vāta's qualities of lightness, exhilaration, and freshness. These are infused into your body just before sunrise and last throughout the day."[95] For evidence of this,

Six Phases of the Day According to Maharishi Āyurveda[96]

Day	*Night*
6 A.M.–10 A.M.—*Kapha*	6 P.M.–10 P.M.—*Kapha*
10 A.M.–2 P.M.—*Pitta*	10 P.M.–2 A.M.—*Pitta*
2 P.M.–6 P.M.—*Vāta*	2 A.M.–6 A.M.—*Vāta*

The times listed vary with season and location.

compare the sense of slowness and heaviness—*kapha* qualities—that can result from waking later in the morning. The main meal of the day is best taken at midday, when the digestive fire, along with the sun, burns brightest, under the domination of the firey *doṣa*, *pitta*, which governs metabolism and distribution of energy. The afternoon *vāta* period can be a time of mental fluidity and efficiency. In the evening one should not fight *kapha's* tendency toward a slow and relaxed pace, and one should go to sleep early, before the resurgence of *pitta* brings about the inclination to wakefulness and activity.

There is another way that time is important to health, not in terms of scheduling daily and seasonal activities, but as regards living within measured time and being either relaxed or suffering from 'time-pressure.' Stress disorders are increasingly recognized in Western medical philosophy. Along with psychological tensions, and physical irritants such as chemical toxins and noise pollution, a sense of time pressure can aggravate and even produce medical problems. In the contemporary world, many persons struggle painfully to accomplish all their tasks within amounts of time that are barely sufficient. Very little unscheduled time is available in modern schedules for rest, recreation, socializing, creative work, and worship. An Āyurvedic approach to life calls us to question the extent to which we sacrifice our health for the sake of our goals and desires, some of which are necessary and worthwhile, and others that can perhaps be relinquished or recast. Āyurvedic living nurtures sensitivity to one's individual requirements for maximal well-being, and can cultivate degrees of energy and vitality beyond what we might have thought possible. This vitality can be used to accomplish goals, but one must put one's health first in order to cultivate vitality.

A suggestion for health-care reform, made by anthropologist and M.D. Melvin Konner, is greater realism (on the part of both patients and providers) about the efficacy of technological solutions for medical problems. He suggests that the public's expectation that high-tech solutions will rescue them from health problems contributes to individuals' irresponsibility for maintaining their own health.[97] In this connection Āyurveda emphasizes prevention, and the individual's responsibility and also *power* to cultivate her or his own health. A person living according to Āyurvedic principles of diet, daily and seasonal routine, and mental attitude is probably less likely to develop conditions such heart disease. Moreover, Āyurveda fosters acute sensitivity to one's health states so that symptoms of incipient illness can be addressed in their early stages.

Āyurveda's notion of equilibrium is dynamic rather than static, and health therefore is not so much a *state*, but a *force:* the power to resist and overcome threats to one's well-being. Embodied life involves a dynamic tension between health and illness; health is not constant well-being, but consists in the power to overcome sickness, to overcome oneself. In his life and thought, Nietzsche valued sickness as well as health, and counted illnesses among "the great stimulants to life."[98] In the tides of illness and health, sickness incites inclination toward life and health, and saying *Yes* to being. The *great health*, Nietzsche says, "one does not merely have but also acquires continually."[99] The *great health* is great enough to encompass illness, so that one can go beyond *accepting* sickness to *affirming* it as a necessary part of life. The Tāntric notion of *śakti*, the dynamic aspect of being, conveys the notion of health as a power: the dynamic force of thriving in one's Self-nature. Thriving entails resistance and overcoming of physical and psychological intrusions to the integrity of one's being. The practice of Yoga serves precisely to cultivate health for overcoming physical and mental intrusions that interfere with the full manifestation of the true Self, which is whole and well. The following chapter, "Classical Yoga as a Religious Therapeutic," applies Āyurvedic concepts of health to reconstruct Yoga's therapeutic paradigm.

Chapter Three

Classical Yoga as a Religious Therapeutic

Among world religious traditions, classical or Pātañjala Yoga is outstanding as a comprehensive system of psychophysical healing and religious liberation. Yoga accounts for the human body/mind and spirit so as to guide practitioners in ethics, health, and progress toward enlightened embodiment. As a religious path, Yoga offers a means for attaining the ultimate soteriological aim: *mokṣa* or freedom from *saṃsāra*, the cycle of rebirth and suffering. Yoga calls liberation *kaivalya*—'independence'—realization of one's true nature—Self-nature as consciousness, independent of materiality (*realization* connoting both 'understanding' and 'achievement'). In this chapter, I cast Yoga's philosophical and religious foundations, along with its eight *aṅgas* ('limbs' or components) of practice, as a system of religious therapeutics with five areas, as shown on the top of the next page.

This model of Yogic religious therapeutics is based on analysis of the *Yoga-sūtras* of Patañjali (c. second/third century C.E.), along with its commentaries the *Yoga-bhāṣya* of Vyāsa (c. fifth/sixth century C.E.) and the *Tattva-vaiśāradī* of Vācaspati Miśra (ninth century C.E.). Since the Yoga teachings are available in broad-ranging texts and detailed commentaries in the original Sanskrit and in translation, access to Yoga's principles, procedures, and potential has been available from ancient times, and will continue to be available in the future. Consonant with the Indian tradition's emphasis on spiritual instruction by a *gūru*, a teacher who is a master of a given tradition, direct guidance in the practice of Yoga is available through the efforts of many teachers in India and throughout the world. Understanding and practice go hand in hand in

Branches of Religious Therapeutics
Based on Classical Yoga's Eight Limbs

Metaphysical and Epistemic Foundations
Yoga's therapeutic paradigm

Soteriology (theory of salvation/ liberation)
Self-realization by healing the afflictions (kleśas)

Value Theory and Ethics
Health and the Good

First limb—Moral self-restraints: Yama
Second limb—Moral commitments: Niyama

Physical Practice
The soteriological role of body and health

Third limb—Postures: Āsana
Fourth limb—Regulation of vital energy through breath: Prāṇāyāma
Fifth limb—Withdrawal of the senses: Pratyāhāra

Cultivation of Consciousness
The polarity of samādhi and vyādhi (illness)

Sixth limb—Concentration: Dhyāna
Seventh limb—Meditation: Dhāraṇā
Eighth limb—Meditative trance: Samādhi

Yoga. Following the path of Yoga requires effort to understand the principles of Yoga, combined with practice of the eight components of Yoga. The *Yoga-bhāṣya* says that practice of the limbs of Yoga destroys unreal cognition and leads to discriminative knowledge [YBh 1.28]. Discriminative knowledge, which distinguishes between materiality and Self-nature as consciousness, is essential for liberation. Discriminative knowledge is a higher form of knowledge than ordinary discursive knowledge. Cultivation of knowledge—by means of self-education such as study of religious and philosophical texts, and the higher knowledge available through meditation—is among Yoga's accessories to attainment of liberation. Like the Indian traditions in general, Yoga considers higher knowledge as the key to liberation, but unique in Yoga is the role it accords the body in the process of attaining it.

MEANINGS AND FORMS OF YOGA

Meanings of 'Yoga'

The word *yoga* is derived from the Sanskrit verbal root √ *yuj*, 'to yoke.' The Indo-European root of *yuj* is √ *yeug-*, which is also the source of the Latin noun *jugum*, yoke, and the English *yoke*.[1] A range of words derives from the Sanskrit *yuj*. Primary meanings of *yuj* are to harness, bind, integrate, unite, or unify. Sanskrit words derived from *yuj* have meanings such as: to meditate, to recollect, to be adapted, joined to, bound by (duty), to be appropriate, and to be logically linked. The derivative noun *yoga* also has a variety of meanings, for instance: the yoking of a team or equipment, union, contact, combination, mixture, connection, relation, performance, employment, use, application, remedy, cure, means, expedient, device, opportunity, undertaking, fitness, propriety, order, succession, effort, exertion, endeavor, zeal, assiduousness, occupation, mental concentration, and meditative abstraction.[2] The great Sanskrit grammarian Pāṇini distinguished the root √ *yuj*, meaning *meditative concentration (yuj samādhau)* from the root √ *yujir*, meaning connecting or yoking (*yujir yoge*).[3] This distinction is made in Vācaspati's *Tattva-vaiśāradī*: "The word 'yoga' is derived from the root *yuj*, to contemplate, and not from the root *yujir*, in which latter case it would mean conjunction" [TV 1.1]. The words 'yoga' and 'religion' share the meaning of yoking: religion is derived from the Latin *ligare*, 'to bind,' 'to bond,' from the Indo-European root √ *leig*, 'to bind.'[4] While a large number of words derived from *yuj* connote yoking or connecting, in classical Yoga, *yuj's* primary meaning is yogic meditative absorption, *yuj samādhau*. However, *yuj* in the sense of 'uniting' is certainly operative in classical Yoga, and refers to unifying one's efforts, integrating one's physiological functions (for instance, by controlling the breath), making one's concentration one-pointed, and overcoming the fragmentation that characterizes ordinary human attention and activity.

Eliade notes that an important meaning of yoga is the effort of yoking one's powers. The purpose of this effort is "to unify the spirit, to do away with the dispersion and automatism that characterize profane consciousness."[5] The effort of self-integration by practice of yoga breaks the bonds keeping *puruṣa*—pure consciousness and the person's true nature—enmeshed in *prakṛti*, the world and the person's mentality and physicality. In devotional forms of yoga, yoking connotes the yoking of the individual with God. Eliade contends that the basic meaning of the verb *yuj*, 'to bind,' presupposes "breaking the 'bonds' that unite the spirit with the world."[6] Despite a variety of applications of *yuj* in the sense of yoking, the ultimate aim of yoga according to the *Yoga-sūtras* is neither the yoking together of the practitioner's aspects nor the joining of the aspirant with the Absolute, but something quite the opposite: *kaivalya*, 'independence.' *Kaivalya* is the liberation of the person's true nature as pure consciousness, independent of material nature, as described in the final verse of the *Yoga-sūtras*:

> *Puruṣārtha śunyānām guṇānām pratiprasavaḥ kaivalyaṃ*
> *svarūpa-pratiṣṭhā vā citi-śakter iti*
>
> Independence (*kaivalya*) is the re-merging of the *guṇas* [constituents of materiality] back into their latent state [as undifferentiated *prakṛti*, materiality], because of their becoming empty of value for the *puruṣa*. Then *puruṣa* is established in its own true nature, in other words, as pure consciousness.
>
> YS 4.34

Liberation in classical Yoga is thus not so much a yoking as a *dissolution* of the bonds of matter, so that consciousness may prevail free of influences of the body, mind, and the material world. Yoking remains integral to the meaning of Yoga in that the practices of Yoga—physical and meditational—entail an effort of one-pointed focusing. One-pointed concentration helps to yoke together the activities of body, breath, senses, and mind, which supports the achievement of non-fragmented mental stillness in the state of *samādhi*.

The most explicit designation of 'yoga' is *yoga-darśana*, the philosophical and religious system of Yoga systematized by Patañjali. The classical Yoga of Patañjali is known as Pātañjala Yoga, Aṣṭāṅga (eight-limbed) Yoga, and Rāja Yoga (the royal yoga, or yoga whereby one becomes master or king, *rāja*, of oneself). Classical Yoga is a synthesis and distillation of a range of traditional Indian techniques of restraint and meditation. In general religio-philosophical terms, 'yoga' designates liberative ascetic techniques and methods of meditation. Eliade discusses two senses of liberation in the Indian tradition:

1. *Transcendental:* transcending the human condition and appropriating another mode of being.
2. *Mystical:* a 'breaking' of the human condition, "a rebirth to a non-conditioned mode of being," which is absolute freedom.[7]

Yogic restraint of ordinary human activities—of vice, near-constant movement of the body, erratic breathing, and chaotic and distractive mental activity—is the means of separating oneself from profane life and aspiring to sacred life.

Yoga in the Vedas, Upaniṣads, and Bhagavadgītā

Yoga in the Vedas

The *Ṛgveda* does not contain references to yoga as a system of spiritual practice. The word 'yoga' in the *Ṛgveda* has meanings such as yoking, connecting, and achieving the unachieved. But the theme of yoking livestock, and the symbolic yoking of powers is a recurring theme. The following hymn uses the metaphor of yoking to liken the work of sacrificial priests to the work of farmers in their fields:

> The inspired poets who know how, harness the plough and stretch the yokes on either side to win favor among the gods.
>
> RV 10:101:4

Agricultural and yoking metaphors abound also in the *Atharvaveda*, which provides a wealth of material concerning Vedic conceptions of healing.

> Homage to the ploughs (*lāṅgala*), homage to thy [wagon-]poles and yokes; let the *kṣetriya* [hereditary-disease-] effacing plant fade the *kṣetriya* away.
>
> AV 2:8.4 (trans. Whitney)

Prāṇa, the vital energy carried by breath, is a fundamental bridge to liberation in yoga, and it is extolled in the *Atharvaveda:*

> Reverence be, O Prāṇa
> to thee coming
> reverence to thee going;
> reverence to thee standing,
> and reverence to thee sitting.
>
> Reverence be to thee, O Prāṇa,
> When thou breathest in (*prānate*)
> Reverence when thou breathest out!
> Reverence be to thee when thou art turned away,
> Reverence to thee when thou art turned hither:
> To thee, entire, reverence be here!
>
> Of thy dear form, O Prāṇa,
> Of thy very dear form,
> Of the healing power that is thine,
> Give unto us, that we may live!
>
> AV 11:4:7–9 (trans. Bloomfield)

Yoga in the Upaniṣads

The *Kaṭha Upaniṣad* provides one of the earliest articulations of yoga, and expresses a central way of conceiving yoga—restraint of the senses—likened to the yoking of "the vicious horses of a chariot driver" [Kaṭh. Up. 3:5]. In this metaphor, the self, *ātman*, rides in a chariot representing the body. The driver is the intelligence or faculty of discriminating wisdom (*buddhi*), and mind (*manas*) is the reins. In this *Upaniṣad* the young man Naciketas receives instruction from Yama, Lord of Death, on the means of attaining Brahman and immortality. Yama teaches that the wise one may transcend joy and sorrow by the yoga-study of what pertains to the self, "set in the secret place [of the heart], dwelling in the depth primeval—by considering him as God" [Kaṭh. Up. 2:12]. Yama instructs that this self is not slain when the body is slain [repeated in *Bhagavadgītā* 2:19–20ā]. Yama describes yoga thus:

> When cease the five [sense-] knowledges
> Together with the mind [*manas*],
> And the intelligence [*buddhi*] stirs not—
> That, they say, is the highest course.
> This they consider as yoga—
> The firm holding back of the senses.
> Then one becomes undistracted.
> Yoga, truly, is the origin and the end.
> Kaṭh. Up. 6:10–11

A six-fold (*ṣaḍaṅga*) yoga is recommended in the *Maitri Upaniṣad.* A beautiful description is given of Brahmā, the One in the sun, in the cooking fire, and in the heart. Realization of the unity of self with the limitless One is attainable by six yogic practices: restraint of the breath (*prāṇāyāmā*), withdrawal of the senses (*pratyāhāra*), meditation (*dhyāna*), concentration (*dhāraṇā*), rational contemplation (*tarka*), and meditative absorption (*samādhi*) [Mait. Up. 6:18]. This sixfold yoga is similar to Pātañjali's eight-fold classical Yoga, which differs only in that classical Yoga begins with moral restraints (*yama*) and observances (*niyama*), and includes posture (*āsana*) but not *tarka* [YS 2.29]. Meditation on the mystical syllable Om is recommended by these *upaniṣads* [Kaṭh. Up. 2:15–17; Mait. Up. 6:21–29ā] as it is in the *Yoga-sūtras.*

In the *Śvetasvatara Upaniṣad*, yoga is prescribed for the realization of Brahman, which pervades all things "as oil in sesame seeds, as butter in cream." [Śvet. Up. 1:15–16]. The *Śvetasvatara* describes the methods and results of yoga practice, indicating how meditative posture, control of the breath, and withdrawal of the senses lead to liberation:

> Holding his body steady with the three [upper parts: head, neck
> and chest] erect,
> And causing the senses with the mind to enter the heart,
> A wise man with the Brahma-boat should cross over
> All the fear-bringing streams.
> Having repressed his breathings here in the body,
> And having his movements checked,
> One should breathe through his nostrils with diminished breath.
> Like the chariot yoked with vicious horses,
> His mind the wise man should restrain undistractedly.
>
> Śvet. Up. 2:8–9

Although liberation is the highest aim of *Upaniṣadic* yoga, the *Upaniṣads* note the health benefits of yoga: sickness, old age, and death are avoided by one "who has obtained a body made out of the fire of yoga" [Śvet. Up. 2:12ā]. Health is named as one of the signs of progress in yoga [Śvet. Up. 2.13]. The *Śvetasvatara* refers to yoga in connection with Sāṃkhya. In the later systematizations of the classical *darśanas*, Sāṃkhya and Yoga are separate but closely related. In the *Śvetasvatara*, Sāṃkhya and Yoga designate two means of attaining knowledge of the absolute: by discriminative knowing and meditative abstraction, respectively [Śvet. Up. 6:13]. In the *Bhagavadgītā*, the major yoga-text preceding Patañjali's systematization of yoga in the *Yoga-sūtras*, Lord Kṛṣṇa teaches Arjuna of a twofold path: "the knowledge-yoga of the Sāṃkhyas" (*jñānayogena sāṃkhyanaṃ*), and the "action-yoga" of the Yogins (*karmayogena yoginam*) [BhG 3:3].

Yoga in the Bhagavadgītā

K. N. Upadhyaya writes that the *Bhagavadgītā* subordinates Sāṃkya's dualism and atheism, along with the methods of yoga, under the theistic and non-dualistic philosophy of Vedanta.[8] In the *Gītā's* Karma Yoga, the yoga of non-detached action, the body is the very instrument of the aspirant's carrying out responsibilities in the world, but with an attitude of non-attachment. While action is necessary in human life, salvation requires *niśkāma karma*, performance of action without attachment to its result, whether pleasant or unpleasant. Kṛṣṇa exhorts the warrior Arjuna: "Fixed in yoga . . . do thy work . . . Yoga is skill in action" [BhG 2:48,50]. Kṛṣṇa's instructing Arjuna to *act*, to carry his duty as a warrior regardless of the consequences—the killing of his kinsmen—exemplifies Karma Yoga's yoking of physical action with emotionally detached understanding. Action is to be performed *in a fully aware and disciplined manner*, with the matter of significance not being the external action and its consequences, but the understanding with which the action is performed. Knowledge permits performance of the action with mental equipoise—without desire or aversion—and this state of equanimity permits and, in part, constitutes the aspirant's liberation and union with God.

'Yoga' in the *Bhagavadgītā* does not have the *Yoga-sūtras'* technical meaning of cessation of the 'turnings' or activities of the mind. The predominant meaning of yoga in the *Gītā* is "disinterested and selfless discharge of one's duty."[9] Upadhyaya identifies a number of other meanings of 'yoga.' In devotional terms, yoga means total surrender to God. In some verses, God's wondrous powers are called *yoga-māyā*. 'Yoga' is also used in the *Gītā* to designate control of the mind and practice of meditation—the meaning of yoga later articulated by Patañjali.[10] Dasgupta suggests that use of the word 'yoga' in the *Bhagavadgītā* has meanings conforming with both *yuj samādhau*, pertaining to meditative concentration, and *yujir yoge*, yoking or connecting. He maintains that both these connotations of yoga serve the *Gītā's* purpose of prescribing a middle path between a meditative life disengaged from worldly activity and the sacrificial action of a vedic worshipper. The *Gītā's* type of yogin both meditates and acts, but he acts more from responsibility than desire, releasing attachment to the pleasant or unpleasant consequences of his actions.[11]

Although Karma Yoga is the predominant form of yoga in the *Gītā*, other paths of yoga are recommended as well. The *Gītā* refers to *āsana* and *prāṇāyāma* [BhG 6:10ff], and gives concise instructions for *Dhyāna Yoga*, the yoga of concentration and meditation. The Gītā offers a choice of yogas for persons of different natures:

> In this world there is a two-fold basis
> Taught anciently by me O blameless One (*Arjuna*).
> The knowledge yoga of the Sāṃkhyas (*jñānayogena sāṃkhyanaṃ*),
> The action-yoga of the yogins (*karmayogena yoginam*).
>
> BhG 3:3

Sāṃkhya theory and yoga practice in the *Gītā* represent Jñāna (knowledge) Yoga and Karma (action) Yoga, respectively. The *Gītā* treats the two paths as having equal value and with the same destination. Bhakti Yoga, the yoga of devotion, can be practiced through either Jñāna or Karma Yoga. Kṛṣṇa instructs:

> By devotion to me he comes to know
> How great and who I am in truth

Then having known me in truth
He enters into me immediately.
BhG 18:55

In all these uses of yoga in the *Bhagavadgītā* is the idea that *knowledge* is the foremost requirement for liberation. The various yogas both require and cultivate understanding that supports discriminative, and hence liberative insight.

Traditions of Yoga Practice

Many forms of yoga are practiced within India's several religio-philosophical currents. These include non-Hindu yogas (Buddhist and Jain), Tāntric yogas, non-systematic and popular forms of yoga, and the classical Yoga of Patañjali. The following discussion identifies major schools of yoga, beginning with yoga in non-Hindu traditions.

In Buddhism, the main problem of Indian soteriology—suffering and emancipation—is treated in part by yogic techniques. Śākyamuni Buddha studied Sāṃkhya doctrines and yoga practice during his six years of seeking enlightenment, and his teachers of these two traditions are named in the early Buddhist texts.[12] A major instance of yogic technique in the Buddha's teaching is *sattipaṭṭhāna*, 'mindfulness' of the body's structure, function, posture, and breathing:

> And how O bhikkus, does a bhikku [monk] dwell observing the body in the body?
>
> Here a bhikku, having gone to a forest, or to the foot of a tree, sits down crosslegged, keeps the body upright and fixes his awareness in the area around the mouth. And with this awareness he breathes in, with this awareness he breathes out. Breathing in a deep breath he understands properly "I am breathing in a deep breath." Breathing out a deep breath he understands properly, "I am breathing out a deep breath."[13]

The Buddhist practice of mindfulness of breathing does not emphasize *physical* action and control of breath as does yogic *prāṇāyāma*, but instead emphasizes *mental* effort, and the gaining of awareness and truth by observing the arising and cessation of physical and mental states. Mindfulness of the body and breath exemplifies Buddhism's emphasis on cultivation of mind and higher knowledge.

Jainism also incorporates yogic practices. For instance, the *Jñānārṇava* of Śubhadra (c. 800 C.E.) discusses postures, regulation of breath, and yogic meditation methods.[14] The Jain scholar Haribhadra (c. 750

C.E.), among his hundreds of other works, wrote treatises on yoga, notably the *Yoga-bindu* and *Dṛṣṭi-samuccāya*. Jainism influenced classical Yoga's ethics, especially its inclusion of the fundamental Jain principle of *ahiṁsā:* non-injury.[15]

Kuṇḍalinī Yoga, part of the Tāntric tradition, uses the esoteric physiology of *cakras*, 'wheels' or energy-centers along the axis of the spine, and *nadīs* or 'channels' (literally 'rivers') through which *prāṇa*, the life-force, circulates. *Kuṇḍalinī* is conceived as cosmic energy, depicted as a snake coiled at the lowest of the *cakras*. The yogin who practices Kuṇḍalinī Yoga aims to redirect his psychospiritual energy, in the form of the feminine principle *Kuṇḍalinī Śakti*, upward through the *cakras* to the crown of the head, where it unites with the masculine principle *Śiva*, resulting in *samādhi*. Yogic practices such as *prāṇāyāma* or control of the breath and vital energy are thought to activate *kuṇḍalinī's* ascent, culminating in attainment of the enlightened consciousness called *samādhi*.[16]

The well-known Haṭha Yoga incorporates doctrines of Kuṇḍalinī Yoga. Haṭha Yoga emphasizes physical purification, *āsana* or postures, and *prāṇāyāma*. Consonant with Tāntrism, Haṭha Yoga regards the perfection of the body as instrumental to attainment of liberation. *Haṭha* means 'force' or 'forceful.' Figuratively, *ha* signifies the heating energy of the sun, and represents inhalation, while *tha* denotes the moon's cooling energy and represents exhalation. Haṭha Yoga's main text, the *Haṭha-yoga-pradīpikā*, presents techniques of activating *kuṇḍalinī* energy for the sake of spiritual progress.[17] Haṭha Yoga is not merely a system of physical cultivation: the *Haṭha-yoga-pradīpikā* integrates physical disciplines with the higher spiritual disciplines of classical or Rāja Yoga, and Haṭha texts present Haṭha Yoga as a means to Rāja Yoga.[18] However, Tantra and Haṭha Yoga are diametrically opposed to classical Yoga in that they consider enlightenment to involve illumination of body as well as consciousness.

The different types of yoga may be considered in terms of six periods in the history of yoga: (1) Proto-Yoga, (2) Pre-classical, (3) Epic, (4) Classical, (5) Post-classic, and (6) Modern yoga. Evidence about the Proto-yoga of the period of the Indus Valley civilization (c. 2600–1500 B.C.E.) exists in archaeological findings such as statues and seals with images of persons in yoga postures, and also references in the first Indian texts, the *Vedas*. Pre-classical yoga consists of the first detailed articulations of yogic practices and meditation in the early *Upaniṣads*, dating from c. 800 B.C.E. Epic yoga (c. 500 B.C.E.–200 C.E.) designates the yoga of the middle *Upaniṣads*, and the great epic the *Mahābhārata*, which includes the revered scripture the *Bhagavadagītā*. For persons of different natures, the *Gītā* offers three yogic paths: *Jñāna Yoga*, the yoga of knowledge, *Karma Yoga*, the yoga of action [BhG 3.3], and *Bhakti Yoga*, the yoga of devotion to the Lord [BhG 18.57]. Jñāna Yoga is cultivation of discriminative knowledge and the use of the mind to free itself from matter and bondage. Karma Yoga is the carrying out of one's earthly and spiritual duties, and serving others, without desire or aversion. Bhakti Yoga, related to both Jñāna Yoga and Karma Yoga, is grounded in adoration of the Lord and offering all one's actions to him.

Classical Yoga (c. second/third century C.E.) denotes the Yoga systematized in *Patañjali's Yoga-sūtras* and expounded by extensive commentaries in subsequent centuries. The *Yoga-sūtras* distill elements of earlier forms of yoga, and systematize an eight-fold program of disciplines culminating in enlightened realization of Self as consciousness—in this life, free of subjugation to embodiment—and after this life, free of a body and its potential rebirth and suffering.

Post-classical yoga (c. 200–1900 C.E.) includes Haṭha Yoga, Tāntric yogas, and the Yoga Upaniṣads. In general, the approximately twenty Yoga Upaniṣads incorporate the subtle physiology of Tantra's Kuṇḍalinī Yoga. The Yoga Upaniṣads do not accept the dualistic metaphysics of classical Yoga, but instead advocate Vedānta, the non-dualistic metaphysics dominating Indian philosophy and religion from the time of the earliest *Upaniṣads* to the present day. Several of the Yoga Upaniṣads list four varieties of yoga:

> Yoga, although one, is according to practice and usage, O Brahman! Differentiated as of various kinds [chief among them are]: Mantra-yoga, Laya-, what is known as Haṭha- and Rāja-yoga.
>
> *Yoga-tattvopaniṣad*, 19

Mantra Yoga aims for dissolution of mind by *mantras*, sacred Sanskrit sounds that are chanted or silently meditated on. *Mantras* are imbued with qualities thought to contribute to meditative awareness and attainment of liberation. Mantra Yoga also employs *prāṇāyāma* and cultivation of the ascent of *kuṇḍalinī*. *Laya Yoga*, the yoga of dissolution [√ *li*, 'to dissolve'], embraces theories and practices of Kuṇḍalinī Yoga. Laya yoga incorporates methods such as meditation on 'the inner sound' (*śadba*), leading to dissolution of mental activity. In Modern yoga, dating from the twentieth century, the work of Śri Aurobindo (1872–1950) is preeminent. His *Pūrna Yoga* or 'Integral Yoga' incorporates elements of Rāja, Haṭha, the *Gītā's* yogas of action, knowledge, and devotion, and the

Tāntric Kuṇḍalinī and Mantra Yogas. Pūrna Yoga offers a spiritual path relevant in the present circumstances of global crisis, and seeks to integrate the quest for individual liberation with humankind's evolutionary destiny.[19]

A MATRIX OF CLASSICAL YOGA AS A RELIGIOUS THERAPEUTIC

Metaphysical and Epistemic Foundations

Yoga's Therapeutic Paradigm

While Yoga is among humanity's greatest religious resources for informing theory and practice in the domain of health, it is a very different relation between health and spirituality that grounds Yoga's higher dimension as a religious therapeutic:

> Yoga physiology or psychology thus takes its direction and significance from the reality which is beyond the body or the psyche. This renders the physio-psychology of yoga sacred. The cultivation of the body or the mind for their own sake is not yoga. The psychic healing of yoga has its centre above the psyche; here the wholeness aspired for is that of holiness.[20]

Yoga upholds a standard of human well being—psychophysical and spiritual—that greatly expands our view of body, health, and human potential. The wholeness that is holiness, the liberation that is healing in its fundamental meaning, is the goal of Yogic religious therapeutics. Yoga's philosophical foundations have a therapeutic orientation whose concern "is not only the diagnosis of the human condition but also the prescription and effecting of a cure that will make man whole."[21]

Yoga's Diagnosis of the Human Condition

Yoga's metaphysics diagnoses the human condition as a state of suffering due to ignorance whose specific form is misidentification of Self with materiality. By understanding the principles that govern nature and the human being, a yogin can "diagnose and thus overcome his fundamental metaphysical illness of 'mis-identification with matter.'"[22] Misery, according to the *Yoga-sūtras*, can and should be prevented [YS 2.16]. The cause of misery is "the conjunction (*saṃyoga*) of the Seer and the Seen" [YS 2.17]. 'Seer' or *draṣṭṛ*, [√ *dṛś* 'to see'] and 'Seen' designate the two forms of primordial Being: *puruṣa* or consciousness—the true Self—and *prakṛti* or materiality—the experienceable world, including one's own body/mind. *Prakṛti* exists for the sake of *puruṣa*; their conjunction serves the *puruṣa's* "recognition of the Self-natures of the two powers" [YS 2.23; SK 21]. Their conjunction ends when it has caused "knowledge of nature of the knower," which is ultimate spiritual freedom [YBh 2.23]. This liberation, called 'independence' (*kaivalya*), is achieved with the individual *puruṣa's* recognition of its Self-nature as consciousness, wholly independent of *prakṛti* and all its material evolutes, including the human mind and body, and everything else in the manifest universe.

The co-presence of *prakṛti* and *puruṣa* engenders the manifest world by disturbing the equilibrium of the *guṇas*, the three main forces of matter/energy comprising all physical things and processes. The *guṇas* are:

1. *Sattva:* purity, illumination and awareness
2. *Rajas:* activity
3. *Tamas:* stability and inertia [SK 12–21]

The *guṇas* are also the three *qualities* characterizing all things. In Yoga, states of mind are described as *sattvic*, *rajasic*, and *tamasic* [TV 1.1, YBh 1.2]. "Mental essence is by nature purity; but it puts on impurity by the taint of disturbing energy (*rajas*) and inertia (*tamas*)" [YBh 1.16]. To say that *puruṣa* is *pure* consciousness is to say that it is awareness entirely independent of *prakṛti* and the *guṇas*. It is awareness without an object external to itself, and without an external object, consciousness can be conscious of itself. The individual *puruṣa* in ordinary human life fails to recognize itself as pure consciousness, because "even though pure [of mental contents], it cognizes by reflecting or imitating the contents of the mind" [YS 2.20]. *Puruṣa* becomes aware of itself by 'reflecting' the *buddhi* or intelligence, which presents objects of knowledge to the *puruṣa*. The *Tattva-vaiśāradī* clarifies with an analogy:

> Although the moon is not as a matter of fact transferred into pure water, it is, so to speak, transferred into it. So also, the power of consciousness, although it is not actually transferred into the *buddhi*, yet it is, so to speak, transferred into it, because it is reflected into it.
>
> TV 2.20

Metaphysics and soteriology are intimately related in classical Yoga. Essential elements of Yoga's metaphysics and soteriology are these reciprocal functions:

1. Discriminative knowledge permitting discernment of the true Self as *puruṣa*.
2. Disentanglement from materiality and from materially oriented desire and aversion that cause suffering and impede self-realization.

Sva-svāmi-śaktyoḥ svarūpopalabdhi-hetuḥ saṃyogaḥ

The purpose of the conjunction (*saṃyoga*) of the master [i.e.,the Seer or experiencer: *puruṣa*] and the experienceable world (*prakṛti*) is the experiencer's recognition of the Self-natures of the two powers.

YS 2.23

Tasya hetur avidyā

The cause [of their conjunction] is ignorance [i.e., *puruṣa's* ignorance of its own real nature].

YS 2.24

Tad-abhvāt saṃyogābhāvo hānaṃ tad dṛśeḥ kaivalyam

By elimination of ignorance, the conjunction of materiality and consciousness is eliminated, and this is the Seer's liberation [*kaivalyam:* 'independence' from *prakṛti*].

YS 2.25

Discernment of *puruṣa* is Yoga's principal soteriological effort. Discernment or discriminative knowledge is called *khyāti* (√ *khyā*, 'to see,' 'to know'). Discriminative knowledge of *puruṣa*, the true Self of each person—which is of the nature of God—conditions attainment of *vairāgya*, 'dispassion' or 'non-attachment' (*vi*, 'without'; √ *raj*, 'to enjoy'). *Vairāgya* is the state of cessation of desire for the *guṇas*.

Tat paraṃ puruṣa-khyāter guṇavaitṛṣṇyam

Dispassion (*vairāgya*) is highest when, owing to discrimination between consciousness and materiality, there is no thirst for the *guṇas* [i.e., no thirst for material objects and experiences, which are formed of *guṇas*, the three basic constituents of matter].

YS 1.16

Cessation of desire for the products of the *guṇas* is equivalent to freedom from entanglement in materiality. Entanglement in materiality results from ignorance of one's Self-nature as independent of materiality. Ignorance, *avidyā*, is the root cause of bondage and suffering. *Puruṣa-khyāti*, discernment of Self, is the remedy for ignorance, and the means of liberation from passion and suffering. Thus *puruṣa-khāyti* is the principle medicament in Yogic religious therapeutics.

The Yogic Remedy

Ignorance, *avidyā* [a, 'not'; √ vid, 'to know'], refers particularly to the Self's ignorance of its true nature. Classical Yoga is an eight-fold remedy to inhibit the activity of the mind, so that the Seer ceases to identify himself with the *vṛttis* or mental experiences, and thus becomes established in his true Self-nature, *sva-rūpa* (YS 1.2–3). The *Tattva-vaiśāradī* explains:

> By the word *svarūpa*, one's own nature, the author excludes the appearance of the calm, the agitated, and the dull, which have been fastened upon it. The nature of the *puruṣa* is consciousness alone, unaffected by the contact (of objects placed alongside it), not the cognitive action of the *buddhi* (the power of intelligence) appearing as calm, etc.
>
> TV 1.3

Because ignorance is considered the source of bondage, liberation requires right knowledge. The importance of knowledge in Yoga is not limited to problems of epistemology, for in Yoga, knowledge—higher or discriminative knowledge—is itself the remedy for the human condition.

Correct judgment (productive of right knowledge), and incorrect judgment (productive of wrong knowledge), along with the other mental processes or *vṛttis*—literally 'turnings' (√ *vṛt*, 'to turn')—are to be stopped by a series of preliminary and meditative practices [YS 1.2]. *Nirodha*, stoppage of the *vṛttis* (√ *rudh* 'to stop', 'to obstruct') embodies Yoga's goal: In the state of *nirodha*, the Seer is established in its own essential and fundamental nature [YS 1.3]. In other states, the Seer identifies with the *vṛttis* [YS 1.4]. Vācaspati gives another analogy for the *puruṣa's* knowing by means of being reflected in *buddhi* (the intelligence), but then mistaking the *buddhi* for itself: the case of one who looks into a dirty mirror, and concludes, "I am dim" [TV 1.4].

The *vṛttis* or processes of the mind occur in five forms:

1. *Pramāna:* Correct judgment (productive of right knowledge) based on perception, inference, or authority
2. *Viparyaya:* Incorrect judgment (productive of wrong knowledge) based on perception, inference, or authority
3. *Vikalpa:* Imagination or conceptualization (mental constructions without corresponding objects) based on images, words, concepts, and/or symbols
4. *Nidrā:* Sleep (including dreaming and dreamless sleep)
5. *Smṛti:* Memory [YS 1.5,6]

Yoga's five-fold classification of *vṛttis* is an elegant account of the innumerable possible instances of human cognition. Right knowledge and wrong knowledge are derived from perception, inference, and/or 'authority' (i.e., a reliable source). In imagination and conceptualization, images, words, ideas, and/or symbols are generated and/or combined in forms or sequences that might not have corresponding forms in the external world. Memory is the mental re-experiencing of previous experiences, physical and/or mental. In *dreaming*, images, meanings, and experiences of the 'subtle body' or 'dream body' occur independently of sensory input, and dream-cognition is non-rational. *Dreamless sleep* is marked by absence of images, meanings, and experiences. Dreamless sleep resembles the one-pointed mind for which Yoga strives, but sleep originates in *tamas* and is therefore contrary to the higher knowledge-states of *samādhi* [TV 1.10]. Complex *vṛttis* may fall in two or more of the five groups, but Yoga holds that any kind of ordinary mental activity can be accounted for according to the five-fold classification. Yoga seeks to suppress states of ordinary knowledge and to cultivate higher knowledge. *Consciousness* that is the person's true nature does not denote the fluctuating states of mind wherein we experience the *vṛttis* of right and wrong cognition, imagination, conceptualization, dreaming, deep sleep, and memory. The mental fluctuations that characterize these states are to be stilled by *abhyāsa*, persistent effort for establishment in *citta-vṛtti-nirodha*, suppression of ordinary mental activity.

Along with *abhyāsa*, the yogin practices *vairagya*, dispassion or non-attachment [YS 1.12–16]. The exercise of *abhāysa* and *vairāgya* lead to development of higher knowledge, permitting realization of the self as pure consciousness. Knowledge in Yoga has two levels:

1. Ordinary knowledge
2. Higher knowledge on which liberation depends:

> *Śrutānumāna-prajñājbhyām anya-viṣayā viśeṣārthatvāt.*
>
> Higher knowledge (*prajñā*) is different from knowledge based on inference or reliable authority, because it has particulars as its object.
>
> YS 1.49

'Particulars' as a designation for objects of higher knowledge connotes the true nature of the things known. Higher knowledge comprehends the infinitesimal constituents that compose the inner nature of objects, and, ultimately, *puruṣa* can comprehend its own nature as *puruṣa*. By contrast, the ordinary means of knowledge (perception, inference, and authority) are capable only of knowing objects as 'generals' [YBh 1.49]. Taimni's commentary on YS 1.49 clarifies the relation between 'particular' and 'general' objects of knowledge. Objects of knowledge are cognized as 'particulars' not because they are known in isolation from other objects of knowledge, but because their particular nature is revealed in their being known within a broader context:

> It is . . . this inability to see things in the background of the whole which is the greatest limitation of intellectual perception [ordinary knowledge], and intuitive perception [higher knowledge] is free from this limitation. In the higher realms of consciousness each object is seen not in isolation but as part of a whole in which all truths, laws and principles have their due place.[23]

Higher knowledge is attainable in *samādhi*, the culmination of Yoga's eight accessories. *Samādhi* itself has a number of successive knowledge-states leading to final liberation. Swami Adidevananda remarks that "The empirical soul is sick as long as it is isolated from the universal spirit."[24] Religious liberation in Yoga overcomes the sickness of this isolation by seeking a desirable form of isolation, *kaivalya:* independence of the Self from body/mind and materiality. The means to this independence is discriminative higher knowledge, attained by systematic cultivation of body/mind and consciousness.

Soteriology

Self-realization by Healing the Afflictions (Kleśas)

Central to the *Yoga-sūtras'* analysis of human suffering is the theory of the *kleśas*, ailments or afflictions (the main one being ignorance) that affect the body and mind, and also affect the person at a more fundamental level of being: the *buddhi* or faculty of knowing. *Buddhi* or intelligence (√ *budh*, 'to know', 'to wake') is the first evolute of *prakṛti* and the faculty most similar to *puruṣa*, because *puruṣa's* power of pure consciousness gives *buddhi* the power to know. In classical Yoga's metaphysics and soteriology, healing at the most fundamental level applies to the *draṣṭṛ*, the Seer or experiencer. The *draṣṭṛ* is the human being inclusive of *buddhi* (the content-free power of intelligence) along with *manas*, the mind (with its contents and personal patterns of meaning-constitution). Also part of *draṣṭṛ* are the body and the sensory-perceptual capacities, which are functions of cooperating physicality and mentality.

Liberation as healing consists in the *draṣṭṛ's* "establishment in its essential nature": *draṣṭuḥ svarūpe'vasthānam* [YS 1.3]. The highest purpose of yoga, says Swami Ramakrishnananda, "is to secure the necessary discipline for the purpose of awakening the spiritual consciousness of man."[25] Non-establishment in Self-nature is a consequence of the Seer's assimilation with the activities of the mind. This non-discrimination of Self from one's mental processes results from 'afflictions' or *kleśas* (√ *klis*, 'to distress, 'to torment'). With the concept of the *kleśas*, the idea of Yoga as a religious therapeutic comes into sharp focus, for Yoga's soteriology is directed to removal of these afflictions, which cause suffering and prevent liberative Self-realization. Dasgupta tells us that Yoga's goal, the transformation of the *buddhi* into its purest state, where it steadily reflects the true nature of *puruṣa*, requires more than knowledge: "a graduated course of practice is necessary."

> This graduated practice should be so arranged that by generating the practice of living higher and better modes of life, and steadying the mind on its subtler states, the habits of ordinary life may be removed.[26]

As in other Indian traditions, liberation in Yoga depends on cultivation of higher knowledge, but Yoga is distinguished by its systematic means of subduing, purifying, and vitalizing the body and body/mind to help bring about attainment of higher stages of consciousness, discriminative wisdom, and liberation. Yoga does not concern itself with the sacred in terms of sacred forces, objects, or rites. Yoga is a theistic tradition. God, known as Īśvara, is free from the influences of *karma* and free of all afflictions or *kleśas* [YS 1.24]. In Īśvara "the seed of omniscience is unsurpassed" [YS 1.25]. He is regarded as the great Teacher, the teacher of the ancient teachers [YS 1.26], who by compassion wishes to teach knowledge and virtue for the liberation of *puruṣas* [YBh 1.25]. Īśvara inspires the aspirant in the effort of self-cultivation. The efficacy of *Īśvara-praṇidhāna*, resignation or devotion to God, is clear from the *Yoga-sūtras'* declaration that *samādhi* may be directly attained by this means [YS 1.23]. For some yogins, surrender to God—devotion to God of all one's actions of mind, speech, and body [YBh 1.23]—is sufficient for attainment of *samādhi*, and the yogin need not begin with the preliminary limbs of Yoga. However, most practitioners need to start at a more elementary level, so Yoga provides a course of disciplines whereby the *kleśas* may be attenuated and liberative knowledge achieved.

The *kleśas* represent varieties of metaphysical illness, afflictions of mistaken attachment to physical and psychophysical aspects of *prakṛti*. There are five *kleśas*:

1. *Avidyā*: Ignorance of the true nature of reality and Self-nature
2. *Asmitā*: Egoism or sense of 'I am'
3. *Rāga*: Attraction accompanying the desirable
4. *Dveṣa*: Repulsion that accompanies the undesirable
5. *Abhiniveśa:* Clinging to life and aversion to death [YS 2.3]

The first *kleśa*, *avidyā*, or ignorance, is the source (literally the 'field,' *kṣetra*) of the others [YS 2.4]. *Avidyā* is the judging of the impure as pure, the non-Self to be the Self and so on [YS 2.5]. Halbfass calls *avidyā* a 'cognitive disease.' *Avidyā* he says, is "a radical misunderstanding of the world and one's true nature. It is essentially self-deception, self-alienation, apparent loss of one's own identity."[27] *Avidyā* is the root of human bondage and suffering, and because the overcoming of ignorance is the crux of liberation in Yoga, the overcoming of the ignorance-based *kleśas* or afflictions is foundational in yogic soteriology. Central to Yogic religious therapeutics is the eradication of ignorance and its derivatives, conceived as afflictions.

The second *kleśa* is *asmitā*, 'I-am-ness' [*asmi*, 'I am']. This *kleśa* is at the root of thinking that one's Self consists in one's faculties of knowing [YS 2.6]. By analogy, the moon sheds light that is not its own, for it reflects the light of the sun. *Asmitā* is the affliction concerning self-identity; it is the mistake of thinking oneself to be the sum of one's mental faculties and their objects. One of the determinants of health is self-identity, and from the standpoint of religious therapeutics, *asmitā*, or impaired self-identity, is a fundamental form of spiritual ill-health. Realization of self-identity is equivalent to liberation in Yoga; it means healing the debilitation and suffering that result from non-establishment in one's essential nature.

In *kaivalya*, *asmitā* is replaced by knowledge of Self as *puruṣa*. The *guṇas* cease to transform and cease to produce modifications that agitate the mind and interfere with Self-knowledge. In *kaivalya*, the purity of the *sattva* and the *puruṣa* are equal [YS 3.56]. *Sattva*, the *guṇa* whose nature is purity and awareness, designates the human's thirteen-part instrument of cognition called *citta*. *Citta* (√ cit, 'to perceive,' 'to know') is composed of *buddhi*, *manas*, and *ahaṃkara* or ego, along with the five sensory faculties (vision, taste, smell, hearing, and touch), and the five organs of action (voice, hands, feet, excretory organs, and sex organs). The *Yogabhāṣya* explains the equilibration of *sattva* with *puruṣa:*

> When the essence of the intelligence (*buddhi*), with the dirt of activity (*rajas*) and dullness and inertia (*tamas*) removed, has the notion of the

> distinctness of the *puruṣa* as its sole remaining object, and all the seeds of the afflictions (*kleśas*) are burnt up, then does it, so to speak, assume a state of purity similar to that of the *puruṣa*.
>
> YBh 3.54

Although *citta* may attain to the purity of *puruṣa* itself, all constituents of the psychophysical person, including the capacities of knowing, are evolutes of *prakṛti.* Equating *citta* with *sattva* or purity in this context means purifying the contents of the mind, so that the individual *puruṣa's* true nature as consciousness manifests without limit. In *kaivalya*, there is cessation of the *guṇas*' transformations, which otherwise produce mental activity. The *guṇas'* transformations cease when they have fulfilled their purpose. The purpose of their combining in myriad ways to produce the manifold universe is, according to Yoga, to permit *puruṣa's* coming to know itself by first knowing the world of *prakṛti.* This is necessary because the embodied *puruṣa,* in order to understand itself as consciousness, initially needs an object of knowledge in order to experience itself as knower. By engaging in progressively deeper modes of yogic meditative knowing, the ultimate natures of *prakṛti* and *puruṣa* are recognized and differentiated, until the *puruṣa* no longer needs engagement with objects of knowledge to experience the process of consciousness that is its nature.

The third and fourth *kleśas*, *rāga*, 'attraction' (√ *raj* 'to enjoy') and *dveṣa*, 'repulsion' (√ *dviṣ* 'to abhor'), both arise because of attachment, that is, the Seer's relation to things and experiences such that he is subject to disturbance of mind due to contact with them [YS 2.7,8]. For a yogin who has attained the goal of self-realization, his sense-organs still make contact with objects of sensation, but when sensations arise they don't agitate the mind or strongly influence the yogin's experience or actions. *Rāga* and *dveṣa* are rooted in ignorance, whose form in this case is failure to distinguish what the *Upaniṣads* call *preya*, pleasure, from *śreya*, the higher good [Kaṭh. Up 2:1–2]. On Yoga's interpretation, *rāga* and *dveṣa* result from attractions and repulsions concerning *prakṛti*, and from the assumption that *prakṛti's* manifestations are ultimate reality.

The fifth and final *kleśa* is *abhiniveśa*, desire for life or aversion to death (√ *abhi*, 'into,' 'toward'; *ni* 'completely,' 'intensely'; √ *viś* 'to enter,' 'to be engrossed'). This affliction produces suffering by causing anxiety about death. Death is ultimately an illusion, for the physical body is an evolute of *prakṛti*, thus not ultimately real. Death is merely the dissolution of the material constituents that compose the body, not the termination of a person's being. In Iyengar's words, yogic practice permits the practitioner to experience "unity in the flow of intelligence, and the current of self-energy. . . . He understands that the current of self, the life-force, active while he is alive, merges with the universe when it leaves his body at death."[28] Aversion to death involves *asmitā* and the mis-identification of body, mind, and senses as the Self. Clinging to life indicates attachment to sensory and cognitive experience, and makes one subject to suffering as a result of separation from pleasant experience and contact with painful experience. Fear of death derives also from attachment to a sense of 'I': "In all living beings exists the self-benediction, 'Would that I were never to cease'" [YBh 2.9].

Along with the five *kleśas* are the nine obstacles or *antarāyāḥ* (√ *antar*, 'between'; √ *ay*, 'to go'):

1. Illness
2. Apathy
3. Doubt and indecision
4. Carelessness
5. Physical and mental laziness
6. Lack of detachment or sensual incontinence
7. Erroneous views
8. Failure to achieve one of Yoga's eight stages
9. Instability in maintaining an achieved stage [YS 1.30]

Illness, *vyādhi*, is first on the list of obstacles and is significant for religious therapeutics because physical illness is specifically identified as interfering with religious progress. Illness and the other obstacles disturb the mind and "turn the aspirant away from the direct path of Yoga" [TV 1.30]. Yoga conceptualizes illness in Āyurvedic terms, as disequilibrium of the body's three constituent *dhātus* or supports [YBh. 1.30; TV 1.30]. Besides the fact that illness can be an obstacle to religious progress, it can be conditioned by mental states, which suggests the hygienic dimension of religious therapeutics in Yoga: the therapeutic value of Yoga for treating psychophysical problems. Swami Adidevananda asserts:

> . . . functional diseases are caused by mental conditions which affect the nervous system. Maladjustment, insecurity, inordinate ambition, fear, frustration and similar tensions affect mental conditions. Spiritual psychology properly used at an early stage could arrest the progress of symptoms. Hence the contribution of Yoga therapeutics should be properly understood.[29]

Swami Adidevananda refers here to Yoga's efficacy for stabilizing mental disturbances, which have adverse effects on the body. There is cooperation between the hygienic and soteriological dimensions of the Yogic religious therapeutic: the religious path of Yoga also has curative power for ordinary psychophysical maladies.

The companions of the obstacles are the 'symptoms of distraction' or *vikṣepas* (*vi*, 'out,' 'asunder'; √ *kṣip*, 'to throw'). The theory of *vikṣepas* accords with Yoga's treatment of mind and body as the primary dimensions of a unitary human entity. The *vikṣepas* are:

1. *Duḥkha:* suffering or mental distress, conditioned by physical or mental factors
2. Despair or depression
3. Unsteadiness of the limbs or body
4. Irregular breathing [YS 1.31]

The *vikṣepas* link the mental with the physical: for instance, mental distress has physical manifestations including shallow, irregular, or labored respiration. Conversely, regulation of the breath can stabilize mental distress. Yoga prescribes a preventative approach to the *vikṣepas:* one-pointed concentration. Rather than permitting one's mind to be fragmented in several directions, one should practice mental concentration on a single object or principle in order to achieve one-pointedness, *ekāgratā*. Curing *vikṣepa* requires the clarification or purification (*prasādaṇa*) of the mind, achievable by cultivating compassion, good cheer, and indifference toward vice; by control of the breath, and other means [YS 1.33–39].

Overcoming the *kleśas* is directly related to achievement of *samādhi*. Subduing the obstacles, *antarāyāḥ*, and eliminating *vikṣepa*, distraction, help develop the concentration necessary for *samādhi*. The *kleśas* contain the reservoir of *karmas* or actions, which produce the myriad experiences in present and future lives [YS 2.12–13]: "the mental field becomes a field for the production of the fruit of actions only when is it watered by the stream of afflictions" [TV 2.13]. When the *kleśas* are destroyed, the vehicle of *karmas* cannot produce fruit because their generative power is destroyed. The *karmas* result in joy or sorrow according to whether their cause is virtue or vice [YS 2.14], but all is misery to persons who have developed *viveka* or the power to discriminate:

> *Pariṇāma-tāpa-saṃskāra-duḥkhair guṇa-vṛtti-virodhāc ca duḥkham eva sarvaṃ vivekinaḥ.*

> All is suffering to discriminating persons, because of pain resulting from change, anxiety, and their subliminal impressions (*saṃskāras*), and because of conflict between the mind's activities (*vṛttis*) and the basic constituents of materiality (*guṇas*).
>
> YS 2.15

Yoga's knowledge-based remedy for the dis/ease of human bondage is the dispersion of ignorance, permitting the dissociation of *puruṣa* and *prakṛti*. This is liberation from the pain of the human condition. How is ignorance to be dispersed? By 'unwavering discriminative knowing': *viveka-khāyti* [YS 2.26]. 'Discriminative knowing' means distinguishing between the experienced world and Self as experiencer. *Viveka-khyāti* in turn produces discriminative knowledge: *prajñā* [YS 2.27].

> *Yogāṅgānuṣṭānād aśuddhi-kṣaye jñāna-dīptir ā viveka khyāteḥ.*
>
> By practice of the limbs of Yoga, which destroy impurity, higher knowledge (*jñāna*) shines forth, reaching up to discriminative knowing (*viveka-khāyti*) [i. e, the power to distinguish Self from materiality].
>
> YS 2.28

Liberative knowledge is not only therapeutic for transcending suffering, it engenders attainment of the human's soteriological potential: "The genuine yogin is a metaphysical doctor, who can not only cure the diseases of the mind, but also who can help us in discovering the possibilities of human consciousness."[30]

On the basis of Yoga's metaphysical view of the person as a psychophysical being at the empirical level, but ultimately an entity of the nature of pure consciousness, health as wholeness and well-being can be ascribed of the person as *puruṣa*, and the term 'healing' may properly denote the process of liberative self-realization. Yoga practice spontaneously promotes physical and psychophysical health. However, more significant about classical Yoga is the way cultivation of the psychophysical person and health contributes to ultimate transcendence of the body/mind.

Value Theory and Ethics

Health and the Good in Yoga

Value theory is an aspect of Yogic religious therapeutics that clearly exhibits the reciprocal relation of Yoga's soteriology and its therapeutic impetus. The highest good in the classical Indian systems "is attained when all impurities are removed and the pure nature of the Self is thoroughly and permanently apprehended."[31] The means to Yoga's highest good, realization of Self as pure consciousness, is stoppage of the activities of the mind, and consequent development of *vivekaja-jñāna*, 'wisdom born of discriminative knowledge.'

> The stream of mind flows both ways; it flows toward good and it flows toward evil. That which flows on to perfect independence (*kaivalya*) down the plane of discriminative knowledge, is named the stream of happiness. That which leads to re-birth and flows down the plane of undiscriminative ignorance, is the stream of sin.
>
> YBh 1.12

The Good in Yoga is that which supports the physical and mental purity necessary for attainment of liberative knowledge. Specifically, Yoga's ethical ideal is *vairāgya*, desirelessness.[32] The mind's tendency toward activity, and the emotions that result, are to be checked by cultivation of *vairāgya* and its companion practice, *abhyāsa:* persistent effort to bring the mind from fragmented activity to a state of "calm one-pointedness and purity" [TV 1.13]. Yoga's ethics emphasize sattvic or pure actions and motives, especially for the sake of calming the mind. *Sattva*, or purity, characterizes health-preserving and health-promoting practices.

Ethics is the foundation of the eight limbs of Yoga, and value theory is integral to religious therapeutics. A person's practice in matters such as diet, sleep, hygiene, exercise, and mental attitude constitute a fabric of daily life, grounded in one's fundamental values (though behavior is consistent with values to varying degrees). Particular physical and mental disciplines incorporate the cultivation of good habits, not just for everyday success, but to serve an aim of progressive self-transformation. The first limb of Pātañjala Yoga is *yama*, embracing five self-restraints, which together constitute the "Great Vow" common to many of the Indian traditions.

First Limb: Moral Self-restraints—Yama

Ahiṁsā, non-injury, the first of the five moral self-restraints, is "not causing injury to any living creature, in any way, at any time" [YBh 2.30]. *Ahiṁsā* is a fundamental ethical principle in Jainism, Hinduism, and Buddhism, and in Yoga it is the foundation of all the other ethical restraints and observances [YBh 2.30]. The restraints pertain to both attitude and action, and non-injury must be practiced toward all sentient beings including oneself. Injury can result in damage to body, mind, projects, and/or property. Injury compromises health, and this is one reason health is of concern in ethics. However, health in Yoga's ethics has significance beyond this. Even though Yoga's aim is spiritual well-being, not mere well-being of body and mind, the well-being that Yoga seeks in ultimate liberation requires self-discipline of body and mind, and that self-discipline contributes to psychophysical health. While Yoga's goal is religious Self-realization, health is regarded as instrumental to this path; therefore, to maintain one's health is an ethical obligation.

Non-healthful practices (such as smoking or inappropriate diet) violate the principle of *ahiṁsā*. Even haste can be a form of violence, for damage to self and/or others may result from rushing to do things without sufficient time. Thus behaviors inciting stress-related syndromes, such as heart disease, aggravated by a sense of time pressure, violate the principle of *ahiṁsā*, so they are contrary to the good, as conceived by Yoga. Physician Larry Dossey notes the modern Western cultural presupposition that linear time is "running out," and our lives with it. He explores the medical implications of human response to time-markers: "the watch, the alarm clock, the morning coffee, and the hundreds of self-inflicted expectations that we build into our daily routine."

> Our sense of time is not only a major determinant in our awareness of pain, it affects our health by influencing the development and course of specific diseases.

Dossey contends that we suffer from "hurry sickness":

> —expressed as heart disease, high blood pressure, or depression of our immune function, leading to an increased susceptibility to infection and cancer. [33]

The metaphysical foundations of Yoga's soteriology counter the distressing and erroneous views that Self is body, and that one's existence ceases at physical death. Yoga's ethical foundation of non-injury is a comprehensive discipline implying freedom from all destructiveness, whether based in ill-will, or in ignorance alone. In terms of personal health maintenance, *ahiṃsā* requires adjustment of attitudes and behavior to prevent direct damage to the body, and avoidance of the mental distress that conditions physical illness.

Satya, truthfulness, the second of the restraints, requires that one neither express non-truths nor omit truths. The purpose of speech is the communication of knowledge. Speech is to be used for the good of others, not to injure, so Yoga prohibits speech that is "deceptive, confused, or barren in knowledge" [YBh 2.30]. As with all yogic ethical principles, along with preserving others' well-being, *satya* serves the purpose of preventing disturbances to the mind. For example, untruthfulness often perpetuates complications engendering distress in self and others. This distress might have manifestations in the form of physical health-problems, as well as generating obstructive karmic consequences. Another reason for truthfulness is to encourage the optimum functioning of *buddhi*, the faculty of discriminative awareness. *Buddhi* allows one to see beyond illusions, and its cultivation requires truthfulness in word, thought, and deed. Truthfulness is a form of ethical integrity, and this means in yogic terms the integration of one's knowledge, values, and action. The practice of truthfulness at the mundane level is requisite for grasping truth at the ultimate level, the truth of *puruṣa* as the ultimate real.

Asteya, non-stealing, refers to any kind of misappropriation, whether of goods, money, or undeserved praise or privilege. Mahātma Gandhi considered any possession of goods beyond those needed for the basic maintenance of life to be a form of theft, as long as there are persons whose basic needs remain unmet.[34] Gandhi's thinking informs the idea of the *healthy communities:* a community's well-being depends in part on each citizen's having access to adequate resources for a wholesome life.

The *Yoga-sūtras'* commentators emphasize that not just theft, but any inclination toward misappropriation must be overcome: "Inasmuch as the functioning of speech and body depend upon the mind, the mental modification is mentioned here as the principle factor" [TV 2.30]. Non-stealing requires development of one's awareness of the subtler forms of misappropriation that may arise in the process of eradicating cruder forms of dishonesty. Consonant with Yoga's prescription for cultivation of consciousness as the means of liberation, truthfulness and non-stealing demonstrate the function of religious therapeutics to perpetuate one's spiritual evolution through purificatory efforts carried out on the stage of the body, but with the aim of purifying the consciousness.

Brahmacarya, the fourth *yama*, is restraint of sensual and especially of sexual enjoyment. Again, this means not merely abstinence from sensual activities and emotions, but eradication of attachment to them, because craving various forms of sensual enjoyment disturbs the mind and causes suffering. The *Yoga-sūtras* list benefits of each of the *yamas*, and the benefit offered for sexual continence is *vīrya:* 'vigor' or heroic life-energy [YS 2.38]. The practitioner sublimates the body for the sake of greater spiritual power: vital energy ordinarily discharged in sexual activity may be rechanneled within a spiritual current. The capability of teaching Yoga to others requires attainment of the power consequent on *brahmacarya* [YBh 2.38].

Aparigraha, non-acquisitiveness, is the fifth and final *yama*. This principle calls for repudiation of all possessions and circumstances not essential for the maintenance of the body. Here again, the health-related warrants underlying this principle are preservation of others' well-being, and elimination of disturbances to the mind. In this context, one should reduce one's concerns about the acquisition, maintenance, and loss of material possessions. Spiritually, non-acquisitiveness breaks the bonds of identification of self with possessions, and the pleasures and pains that go with gaining, having, and losing them.

Second Limb: Moral Commitments—Niyama

Śauca, purity, is of utmost importance in Yoga. Purity means physical cleanliness, mental clarity, and moral rightness. Purity in physical cleanliness—internal and external—is achieved by bathing, and by various 'washings' with air in *prāṇāyāma*, and with water and other means in yogic physical purification techniques.[35] Especially important is "washing away the impurities of the mind" [YBh 2.32]. In ordinary human life, impurity is pervasive, and yogic religious therapeutics replace impure physical and mental materials and actions with increasingly pure ones. What is purity, in a yogic sense? The *guṇa* called *sattva* is purity itself. To purify is to support the predomination of *sattva*, the *guṇa* that is the nature of *buddhi*, the power of intelligence. Functionally, something is pure to the extent that it permits the manifestation of an entity's true nature as *puruṣa*, and impure to the extent that it supports entanglement in *prakṛti*, thus impeding the expression of *puruṣa*.

Purity may be understood in its various applications in terms of the three 'bodies' or 'vehicles' composing the person [VC 87–97]. The gross body is made pure particularly by consumption of sattvic food and drink. The *Bhagavadgītā* classifies types of foods according to the three *guṇas* [BhG 17.7–10]. Sattvic food is light, fresh, and nourishing, and includes grains, seeds, fruit, vegetables, and dairy foods, according to their agreeability to a given person's constitution. Sattvic food promotes health, *ārogya* [BhG 17.8]. The stimulating rajasic foods are very hot, bitter, sour, dry, salty, or excessively spiced, and include beverages containing caffeine. Rajasic foods, the *Gītā* says, cause pain and sickness, *āmaya* [BhG 17.9]. Tamasic foods promote inertia and restrict *prāṇa*, the vital life-energy. Tamasic foods include flesh, alcohol, and fermented foods such as vinegar, and foods of any type that are stale or spoiled.[36] R. S. Khare identifies two main Hindu formulations of the relationship of food, Self, and ultimate reality. The *Gītā* represents the position that

"You eat what you are." In other words, dietary preferences reflect a person's nature as sattvic, rajasic, or tamasic.

> The second formulation bases itself on the upaniṣadic instruction—pure nourishment leads to pure mind or nature (*ahāraśuddhau sattvaśuddhi*; see Hume, *Principal Upaniṣads*, 1985, 262). As a corollary therefore, a healthy body is considered to be a byproduct of discriminating and controlled nourishment. Diseases follow from flaws—moral, mental, and physical.[37]

Khare's analysis corroborates the idea of religious therapeutics in the context of Indian gastrosemantics. He refers to the work of Hindu holy persons who dispense healing foods and herbs:

> Over time, they acquire the dual therapeutic-spiritual authority which even vaidyas (or "doctors") cannot dispute. . . . If they are known to cure incurable bodily diseases, they also treat the "disease" of transmigration—*saṃsāra* (also called *bhavaroga*).[38]

Yoga philosophy holds that the very material of the physical body is composed of the *guṇas* obtained in the diet, and consonant with the upaniṣadic dietary principle, "You are what you eat," Yoga's goal of dietary purification is the actual replacement of the body's coarser material with more refined material.

The subtle body is purified by replacing disturbed thoughts and emotions with more refined and subtle ones. Purification is a self-perpetuating process, because the more pure body and mind become, the more they incline toward pure substances, thoughts, and emotions. An important purificatory practice for the subtle vehicle is the use of *mantras*. *Mantras* are sacred sounds, the primordial one being *AUM* (*Om*), the designator of Īśvara [YS 1.27]. The vibrations experienced in producing or hearing or meditating on *mantras* permit an influx of spiritual force, which over time tend to remove obscurity from the subtle body. In addition to their vibratory powers, some *mantras* have meanings that are purificatory insofar as the practitioner's ignorance is dispelled by them.

The causal or karmic body is the locus of karmic activity; it is the body constituted of all the consequences—good and bad—of a person's actions in the present life and prior ones. Purification in the domain of the causal or karmic body means burning up the residue of past actions so that no new consequences result, and so that no new actions are taken productive of further karmic results. For a yogin, *karmas* are "neither white nor black" [YS 4.7], that is, neither good nor evil. They are not 'good,' for the yogin gives up the fruit of action, and not 'bad,' because he does not perform actions [YBh. 4.7]. Yoga's treatment of the mental and the physical as reciprocally related dimensions of the unitary person is evident in the range of applications of *śauca*. Purity is a necessary condition for psychophysical health, and the spiritual purity supported by physical health is in turn instrumental for the ultimate healing of liberation.

Saṃtoṣa, the second element of *niyama*, means contentment, "the absence of desire to obtain more of the necessities of life than one already possesses" (YBh 2.32). *Saṃtoṣa* means absence of greed, resulting in calmness and serenity regardless of external or internal circumstances. Such contentment is one of the determinants of mental health. Contentment is a means to the end of mental equanimity, the state wherein mind is without disturbance, and Self-nature can be realized. To practice contentment is more than stilling mental disturbances as they intrude; it entails preventing their arising.

Tapas, translated as austerity, self-discipline, or purification, "consists in endurance of the pairs of opposites" such as heat and cold, and the desire to eat [YBh 2.32]. The verb √ *tap* means 'to heat,' and *tapas* may be likened to the purification of metals by intense heat so that the dross is burned away and the pure metal remains. *Tapas* involves fasting and observance of various vows, such as the vow of silence. *Tapas* may also be performed by practicing *prāṇāyāma*. *Tapas* ordinarily involves self-discipline of the physical body, with the intention of weakening the association of the physical body with consciousness, making possible an awareness of the body as 'not-self.' Impurity leads to illness—physical, mental, and spiritual—and *tapas* represents practices that not only remove impurities but contribute to endurance and non-susceptibility to help make the body/mind a fit vehicle for the spiritual journey.

Svādhāya means self-education. *Adhyāya* means study or education; its verbal root is √ *dhī*, 'to think.' The prefix *sva*, 'self,' underscores the *sādhaka's* individual effort toward self-realization by exerting his or her intelligence. *Svādhāya* includes study of scriptures, pondering of religious and philosophical questions, recitation of mantras, and, ultimately, leaving the texts and disciplines behind and gaining knowledge from within oneself.

Īśvara-praṇidhāna, surrender to Īśvara or God, means "the doing of all actions to fulfill the purpose of the Great Teacher" [YBh 2.32]. Dedicating oneself to the will of God destroys the ego through merging the individual with the sacred, the all-embracing consciousness. This *niyama* is embodied in the *Bhagavadgītā's* prescriptions of *niśkāma karma*, acting without desire, and Karma Yoga, the yoga of action: acting to carry out one's responsibility without attachment to the good or bad results of the action, thus serving divine will rather than one's own. Surrender to Īśvara may also take the form of Bhakti Yoga, the yoga of devotion, where union is achieved through love of God. Whether accomplished by the yoga of action or the yoga of devotion, surrender to God produces dissolution of the 'I' or *asmitā* and thus supports *samādhi*, enlightened consciousness devoid of the traps of egoism.

Yoga's prescriptions for reconditioning the body and mind widen the range of their adaptability, making the practitioner's body, mind, and senses less vulnerable to the "pairs of opposites" (e.g., heat and cold, joy and sorrow) that keep one mired in physicality and separated from one's true nature. Crawford notes that matter is not equated with evil in Yoga, for "both the design and function of *prakṛti* are aimed at the liberation of *puruṣa*."[39] Yet one of Yoga's vital concerns is self-understanding in relation to the material aspects of oneself and the world. The eight limbs of Yoga map out a progressive journey of subduing one's subjugation to materiality and its accompanying physical distractions, mental fragmentation, and emotional ups and downs. The foundation of Yoga as a religious therapeutic is a system of ethics that governs relations among persons, but whose basis is the individual's mastery of physical and mental dispositions and actions that interfere with stilling the mind.

Physical Practice

The Soteriological Role of Body and Health in Yoga

The soteriological role of the body in Yoga concerns refining, disciplining, and utilizing the body/mind complex to make it a less obstructive factor and more suitable instrument for the spirit's purer expression of itself.

> Spiritual awareness is invariably preceded by physical health and mental hygiene. The latter are the means for the former. So Yoga may be described as a science of spiritual healing. Yoga methods are superior to other methods in so far as they take man in his totality and do not deal with him superficially.[40]

Health of the body and non-attachment to physicality are cultivated for spiritual progress. Practice of Yoga's ethics, psychophysical disciplines, and procedures for meditation spontaneously promote health, but health is a help to spiritual attainment, and is not itself the goal. The physically based practices of yoga are *āsana* or postures, *prāṇāyāma* or control of vital energy by control of breath, and *pratyāhāra*, withdrawal of the senses. Their chief purpose is preparation of the practitioner for Yoga's final three limbs: concentration, meditation, and the higher consciousness of *samādhi*, which we may translate as 'meditative trance.' The key textual source for study of the external limbs of Yoga is Section Two of the *Yoga-sūtras*, *Sādhana-pāda*. *Sādhana* means 'practice,' 'discipline,' or 'means,' and pertains to practice conducive to the attainment of a goal. Its verbal root is *sadh*, 'to accomplish one's goal,' or 'to hit the target' (also the root of *sādhu*, 'holy man,' one who has achieved the aim). The term *sādhaka* refers to a practitioner, a person who undertakes *sādhana* with the purpose of accomplishing an aim, particularly a spiritual aim. Practice of the whole system of eight-fold Yoga is a *sādhana*, but the term *sādhana* can also refer to a particular practice, such as *āsana*.

Third Limb: Postures—Āsana

Āsana (√ *as*, 'to sit') literally means 'sitting' or 'posture.' Only three of the 196 verses of the *Yoga-sūtras* deal with *āsana*.[41] According to Patañjali, the two criteria for proper performance of postures are that they must be steady (*sthira*) and comfortable (*sukham*) [YS 2.46]. The main purpose of *āsana* is to render the physical body non-disturbing to the mind. This has two primary applications. First, in the stages of meditation of the sixth, seventh, and eighth limbs, the mind's activity is successively restricted, and the body is to remain as externally motionless and internally undistracted as possible. The *āsanas* are designed so that the body may feel comfortable and thus for the duration of meditation be of no concern to the mind, so that the *sādhaka's* consciousness may take priority in his awareness and being. *Āsana's* other main function is to develop the body's endurance and equilibrium. Practice of *āsana* helps one develop non-attachment to the body and objects of physical enjoyment, and increased capacity for carrying out the responsibilities of life and the yogic path.

Āsana's role in meditation exemplifies the soteriological role of the body in Yoga: physical well-being is not cultivated as an end in itself, but because refined awareness and discipline of one's physical nature contribute to transcending the limitations of physicality and the ignorance and suffering that attend it. Yoga accounts for the human condition from its lowest state of being mired in ignorance and evil, to its highest potential state: realization of its nature as pure consciousness. Yoga is a practical system and provides for individuals to begin the path of Yoga at their own level of awareness and functioning. For most persons, self-understanding and action is deeply rooted in physicality, and Yoga makes use of this fact by providing physical disciplines effective for gaining mastery and insight with respect to one's Self-nature.

Performance of *āsana* also develops endurance and equilibrium. Endurance is the power to act in a sustained way, being 'fit' or suited to tasks requiring a continued application of effort and concentration. Endurance refers to an individual's sustained functioning without symptoms of debilitation. The term 'endurance' may suggest a person's application of sustained energy directed toward an aim, whether religious or, for instance, athletic. Equilibrium is another significant determinant of health, and this concept is applicable at a number of levels of functioning. In Āyurvedic medicine, equilibrium signifies a health-supporting relation among the *doṣas*. In physiological terms, equilibrium pertains to conditions such as coordinated nervous and muscular control for maintaining the body's posture, and commensurate intake and output of substances by organs and systems. Psychological equilibrium concerns a person's resilience in maintaining a stable affective state, and functioning effectively when confronted with difficulties. Equilibrium is treated in the *Yoga-sūtras* in terms of 'the pairs of opposites.' The mastering of *āsana* produces resistance to assault by the pairs of opposites, or *dvandvas* [YS 2.47–48]. The *dvandvas*, such as heat and cold, pleasure and pain, may be experienced physically and/or mentally, and they disturb the mind's equilibrium. Reducing one's distraction by the *dvandvas* is integral to stilling the *vṛttis* or activities of the mind.

Āsana is mastered by 'relaxation of effort' and 'meditation on the infinite': *ananta* [YS 2.47]. *Ananta* literally means without end (*a*, 'not'; *anṭa*, 'end') and can refer to Īśvara. Relaxation of effort means ceasing to give mental attention to maintenance of a posture, so that the body is undisturbed and the conscious mind is gradually freed from agitation by physical sensation. Relaxation is a determinant of health, both intrinsically, as a state of relative freedom from unpleasant tension, and instrumentally, as a capacity of resilience that helps one tolerate and recover from the strain of effort.

In *āsana* the body must become able to maintain physical stability and to counter deviation from its position during meditation. Iyengar discusses *āsana's* unifying functions as follows:

> Though the practitioner is a subject and the *āsana* the object, the *āsana* should become the subject and the doer the object, so that sooner or later the doer, the instrument (the body) and the *āsana* become one. . . .

> The whole body is involved in this process, with the senses, mind, intelligence, consciousness and self.[42]

He describes *āsana's* two aspects as pose and repose. Posing is acting to arrange the body in a particular posture. Reposing is reflecting on the pose and readjusting it:

> . . . so that the various limbs and parts of the body are positioned in their places in a proper order and feel rested and soothed, and the mind experiences the tranquility and calmness of bones, joints, muscles, fibres, and cells.[43]

Health of the physical body at the level of the 'body (literally, 'sheath') of breath or life-force'—*prāṇamaya kośa*—is, according to Iyengar, gained at the level of the cells, which he regards as possessing memory and intelligence. To perform *āsanas* properly entails the elimination of dualities between body and mind, mind and *puruṣa*. Through the health of the body, the mind and *puruṣa* are brought closer. The purpose of *āsana* is "to lead the mind from attachment to the body towards the light of the soul."[44] In Iyengar's "Tree of Yoga" *āsana* is symbolized by branches in their various positions. The roots of the tree represent *yama* (the moral self-restraints), and the trunk is *niyama* (the moral commitments). The fourth part of Yoga is expansion of the vital energy, *prāṇa,* through control of the breath. *Prāṇāyāma* is represented by the leaves of the tree, which permit the tree's respiration.[45]

Swami Vivekananda (1863–1902), who was instrumental in introducing Hinduism to the West, gives brief consideration to *āsana* in his lectures on classical or Rāja-Yoga. He recommends that one choose a meditation posture one can maintain for a long time, with the spinal column held straight and free, and the weight of the body supported by the ribs. Vivekananda compares *āsana* in classical Yoga to Haṭha Yoga, which emphasizes the health and strength of the physical body. Health in Rāja Yoga, he reminds us, is only a means to an end, since an unhealthy or unfit body is the first of the obstructions to Yoga practice.[46]

The effects of *āsana* are subtle and powerful. Practice of *āsana* inclines one toward more wholesome pursuits. The awareness and vitality granted by *āsana* influence a person's choices in avoiding debilitating influences in a range of contexts, for example, unethical dealings, impure foods, and the extremes of sloth or excessive activity and stress. Cultivation of good habits, which in turn improve one's future dispositions, is well exemplified by *āsana's* soteriological role for the Yogin. Another result of the regular practice of *āsana* is a more acute awareness of one's body and its functioning. Daily *āsana* provides an opportunity to take account of physical strengths and weaknesses, flexibility, and areas of impeded energy. Throughout the day, one may spontaneously notice her posture and circulation, and adjust the body to a closer approximation of the excellent posture and circulation promoted during the actual performance of *āsana*. Circulation refers not just to physical substances such as blood, oxygen, lymph, and chyle, but to *prāṇa*, the vital energy of the cosmos and the living organism. *Āsana* "clears the nervous system, causes the energy to flow in the system without obstruction and ensures an even distribution of that energy during *prāṇāyāma*."[47] The practice of Yoga is engaged not only while one does *āsana*, *prāṇāyāma*, and meditation, but is a constant commitment. *Āsana* serves to refine one's physical nature to be increasingly attuned with the subtle prāṇic force in oneself, which may be likened to a current within the great ocean of conscious energy that is *puruṣa*.

The soteriological role of the body in Yoga is evident in *āsana's* power as a means for one to appropriate and integrate the conditions of his physical being. This is consonant with Deutsch's presentation of the body as an 'achievement concept,' and personhood as a matter of integration and achievement.[48] In Yoga, the selfhood that the *sādhaka* seeks to achieve is not that of self as embodied person, but of that of one's true nature as consciousness. *Āsana* helps the physical body to reveal and awaken the power of consciousness that infuses the material body, thus potentiating the discrimination of *puruṣa* from *prakṛti*.

In addition to its soteriological efficacy, *āsana* has physically therapeutic applications. Āyurvedic physician Vasant Lad has shown that Yoga has value for both prevention and cure of illness:

> Yoga brings man to the natural state of tranquility which is equilibrium. Thus, yogic exercises have both preventive and curative value. Yogic practices help to bring natural order and balance to the neuro-hormones and the metabolism and thus provide fortification against stress. Yogic practices for the treatment of stress and stress-related disorders (such as hypertension, diabetes, asthma and obesity) are remarkably effective.[49]

Lad lists appropriate *āsana*s for various ailments,[50] as does Iyengar in *Light on Yoga*.[51] An article on *āsana* in the journal *Brahmavadin* discusses the importance of health for the achievement of spiritual aspirations and identifies the joint medical and soteriological function of *āsana:*

> The aim of the healing art is twofold inasmuch as it renders the body impenetrable to disease from the outside and at the same time it does

> not allow the vital currents in the body to leak out and get exhausted. The postures may be said to be helpful in both these directions.[52]

The cooperation of healing and salvation by yogic means is warranted from earliest times in the Hindu tradition: The *Atharva-veda* says, "With Yoga I drive far away the sin of thy soul and the disease of thy body" [AV 6:91.1].

Fourth Limb: Regulation of Vital Energy Through Breath—Prāṇāyāma

Practice of various *āsanas,* provided that they are suitable *āsanas* for a particular person, and correctly performed, contributes to regulation of the vital energy, *prāṇa,* and so leads naturally to proper performance of the next stage of Yoga, *prāṇāyāma. Patañjali* defines *prāṇāyāma* as "the cessation of the motion of inhalation and exhalation" [YS 2.49–50].[53] The word *prāṇa* is derived from the verbal root √ *an,* 'to breathe,' while the root √ *pra,* means 'to fill.' *Prāṇa* means breath, but, more important, it means vital energy, life-force, spirit, and power. The word *prāṇāyāma* is composed of *prāṇa* and *ayama,* 'extending' or 'controlling' √ *yam,* 'to reach'). Vivekananda explains that while *prāṇa* is often taken to mean breath, it is actually the energy of the cosmos, and the energy in each living body. The motion of the lungs is the most visible manifestation of *prāṇa,* and control of the breath is the most direct means of gaining awareness and control of the *prāṇa* in oneself.[54]

According to Vivekananda, *prāṇa* is the origin of all energy, "the infinite, omnipresent manifesting power of this universe."[55] In the domain of physics, *prāṇa* manifests as forces such as motion, gravitation, and magnetism. In the human body, "It is the *prāṇa* manifesting as the actions of the body, as the nerve currents, as thought force."[56] To get hold of the subtle vibration of *prāṇa* in oneself is the means, Vivekananda says, of grasping the whole of *prāṇa* that is the energy source of the whole universe, and into which everything resolves at the end of each cycle of time.[57]

Prāṇa and its manifestation as breath is crucial for inquiry into body and religiousness. The English word spirit derives from the Latin, *spīrāre,* 'to breathe.'[58] The word 'spirit' connotes vital breath, as does the Sanskrit *prāṇa.* Like *prāṇa,* 'spirit' suggests incorporeality, and the principle that gives life to the body. As the life-principle, and in its connotation of immateriality, spirit is aligned with divine entities and with the sacred. The 'spiritual' is the sacred; human 'inspiration,' the drawing of breath, is the constant sign of our participation in the sacred power of the universe.

In Western concepts of person, 'spirit' can mean a mediating force between a person's body and soul. In physiological terms, breath is subject to both voluntary and involuntary control. Breathing prevails in our waking, sleeping, and even unconscious states, yet it may be controlled in its depth, timing, and quality. Yoga identifies breath as an effective psychophysiological bridge to gaining control of the movement of the subtle energy, *prāṇa*—the energy funding the mind's activities—and thus to achievement of Yoga's goal, *citta-vṛtti-nirodha:* calming the *vṛttis*, or 'turnings' of the mind.

To illustrate the function of *prāṇāyāma*, Swami Vivekananda tells a parable about a king's minister whom the king imprisoned in a high tower. The minister asked his wife to bring to the tower a beetle, some honey, and some silk thread, pack thread or string, twine, and rope.

> The husband ordered her to attach the silken thread firmly to the beetle, then to smear its horns with a drop of honey, and to set it free on the wall of the tower, with its head pointing upwards. She obeyed all these instructions, and the beetle started on its long journey. Smelling the honey ahead it crept slowly onwards, in the hope of reaching the honey, until at last it reached the top of the tower, when the minister grabbed the beetle and got possession of the silken thread. He told his wife to tie the other end to the pack thread, and after he had drawn up the pack thread, he repeated the process with the stout twine, and lastly with the rope. The rest was easy. The minister descended from the tower by means of the rope, and made his escape. In this body of ours the breath motion is the "silken thread"; by laying hold of and learning to control it we grasp the pack thread of the nerve currents, and from those the stout twine of our thoughts, and lastly the rope of *prāṇa*, controlling which we reach freedom.[59]

In the most basic terms, *prāṇāyāma* involves stopping the breath for some amount of time between inhalation and exhalation. Ordinary breathing is erratic, varying with an individual's mental and physical states. *Prāṇāyāma* serves to steady the mind and nerve currents by controlling the breath, thus controlling the energy of the body/mind system.

> To bring under the influence of the will both the physical and mental conditions by introducing rhythm into them is the method of the exercise of *prāṇāyāma.*[60]

Iyengar explains: "Normally the breath is unrestrained and irregular. Observing these variations, and conditioning the mind to control the inflow, outflow, and retention of the breath in a regular, rhythmic pattern, is *prāṇāyāma.*"[61] The technique of stilling the breath is called *kumbhaka*. *Kumbha* means 'jar,' 'vessel,' or 'receptacle': the body and particularly the lungs are the receptacle for *prāṇa*. In *puraka* (√ *pūr*, 'to fill'), the lungs are filled with air and the breath is held. In *recaka* (√ *rik*, 'to empty'), air is exhaled from the lungs and breathing is suspended [TV 2.49].

> *Bāhyābhyantara-stambha-vṛttir deśakāla-saṃhkyābhiḥ paridṛṣṭo dīrgha-sūkṣmaḥ.*
>
> *Prāṇāyāma's* modifications—external [cessation of breath prior to inhalation], internal [cessation of breath prior to exhalation], and restrained [restraint of both of these by a single effort]—are regulated by place, time, and number, thus becoming progressively prolonged and subtle.
>
> YS 2.50

Puraka is 'external' *prāṇāyāma*, and *recaka* is 'internal.' 'Restrained' means cessation of both of these 'by a single effort' [YBh 2.50]. *Prāṇāyāma's* 'regulation by place' pertains to directing *prāṇa* to particular parts of the body. 'Regulation by time' refers to ratios of time for the three parts of *prāṇāyāma:* inhalation, exhalation, and suspension of breath. Various techniques and ratios of inhalation, exhalation, and retention of breath constitute the different forms of *prāṇāyāma*, and these variations serve different purposes for individual practitioners.[62] Gradually *prāṇāyāma* becomes more "prolonged and subtle" [YS 2.50]. Vācaspati explains:

> This *prāṇāyāma* becomes of long duration when it takes up greater space [measured by the effect of the breath outside the body and the sensation of it within the body] and time. . . . It is subtle, because it is known by a very subtle trance (*samādhi*), not because it becomes weak.
>
> TV 2.50

The yogin's acute awareness and command of *prāṇa* may progress beyond the external, internal, and restrained forms, to the fourth and highest form of *prāṇāyāma*, by which, Patañjali says, "the covering of light is dissolved" [YS 2.51–52]. This covering is "that by which the *sattva* of the thinking substance is covered, in other words, hindrances and evil" [TV 2.52].

Prāṇāyāma purifies the *nadīs* or energy channels of the body, and ultimately helps to purify the mind of its restless activity, confusion, and bondage to matter. I. K. Taimni, in his translation of the *Yoga-sūtras*, gives the following simile to convey the effects of one form of *prāṇāyāma*, alternate nostril breathing (Anuloma Viloma), on the prāṇic currents in the *prāṇamaya-kośa* or body of breath:

> When we breathe normally the prāṇic currents follow their natural course. When we breathe alternately through the two nostrils their normal flow is disturbed in some way. The effect may be likened to the flow

> of water in a pipe. When the water is flowing in one direction placidly, silt and other things may be deposited at the bottom and are not disturbed to any marked extent by the water. But try to force the water in opposite directions alternately and you at once disturb the deposit, and if the process is continued long enough the pipe gets cleaned ultimately.[63]

Each of the five *prāṇas* or *vāyus*, vital 'breaths,' 'airs,' or 'forces,' is responsible for functions within a particular region of the body, as shown in the table below. *Apāna vāyu,* the 'downward air' also has the meaning of displaced *prāṇa*. When a person is unsteady, confused, or otherwise disturbed, his *prāṇa* is not confined within him, but is scattered beyond his body. A yogin, on the other hand, is "one whose *prāṇa* is within the body."[64] *Apāna vāyu* can also refer to impurities in the body, which can be reduced at the subtle level of prāṇic energy by the cleansing force of *prāṇāyāma*. Invoking the *Haṭha Yoga Pradīpikā's* image of the center of the body as 'the seat-of-fire' [HYP 3.65–66], Desikachar maintains that defilements in the body interfere with *prāṇa* entering the body. On inhalation, *prāṇa* in the air surrounding the body is drawn into the body where it meets the *apāna* or impure air. On exhalation, the *apāna* moves toward the *prāṇa*. The powers of respiration, digestion, and metabolism in the center of the body are likened to flames, and the energy of *prāṇa* in

The Five Vāyus *or Vital Forces*

Udāna Vāyu: Rising Air
  Operates between throat and top of head, responsible for processes including speech.

Prāṇa Vāyu: Vital Air
  Operates between throat and navel, controls, respiration and circulation.

Samāna Vāyu: Equal Air (carries nutriment, etc., equally to all parts of body)
  Operates between navel and heart; its main responsibility is control of digestion.

Vyāna Vāyu: Pervading Air
  Operates throughout the whole body, assisting other *vāyus*. It controls body movement, gross nerves, and the subtle *nādīs* or energy channels.

Apāna Vāyu: Downward Air
  Operates from navel to soles of feet; controls excretion, and sexual and reproductive functions.

YBh 3.38[65]

this region in effect 'burns' the defiling *apāna* upon inhalation. Equally important is the expulsion of this burnt residue, achieved by exhalation. The diverse patterns of inhalation, exhalation, and retention of breath maximize *prāṇāyāma's* purificatory functions.[66] In classical Yoga, *prāṇāyāma* demonstrates the soteriological role of the body by its capacity to increase the health and vitality of the body, and to reduce the *citta-vṛttis* or 'mind-waves,' preparing the *sādhaka* for attainment of the higher states of consciousness in the final three 'inner limbs' of Yoga, which are progressively deeper stages of meditation.

Prāṇa is integral to Yoga's understanding of health. Disease can be characterized in terms of disturbance in the balance of *prāṇa* in the body, "so the best way for keeping the body free from disease is by preserving an even circulation of *prāṇa*."[67] *Prāṇāyāma's* chief purpose is to gain control of *prāṇa* for the sake of attaining enlightened consciousness. *Prāṇāyāma* concentrates *prāṇa* within the body by stilling the mind through regulating the *prāṇa*-carrying breath. Reciprocally, yogic mental culture produces greater mental clarity, thereby reducing distress, reflected in regulation of the operations of breath and *prāṇa* in the body. Eliade writes that *prāṇāyāma* stabilizes physiological unevenness, and is the gateway to a deeper mode of being:

> *Prāṇāyāma*, we should say, is an attention directed on one's organic life, a knowledge through action, a calm and lucid entrance into the very essence of life.[68]

Fifth Limb: Withdrawal of the Senses—Pratyāhāra

Pratyāhāra is the transition between the first four preparatory components of Yoga and the final three meditative components. The word is composed of the adjective *prati*, 'against,' 'return,' or 'withdrawal,' and *hara*, 'bearing' or 'bringing' (√ *hri*, 'to hold,' 'to carry'). A technical term in Yoga, *pratyāhāra* refers specifically to withdrawal of the senses from their objects. Desikachar suggests a figurative way to interpret the term: *āhāra* means 'food,' so *pratyāhāra* suggests "withdrawing from that on which we are feeding."[69]

> *Sva-viṣayāsaṃprayoge citta-svarūpānukāra ivendriyāṇām pratyāhāraḥ.*
> Withdrawal of the senses (*pratyāhāra*) is that in which the senses, by not contacting their objects, imitate, so to speak, the nature of the mind.
> YS 2.54

> *Tataḥ paramā vaśyatendriyāṇām.*
> From this is gained ultimate mastery over the senses.
> YS 2.55

The *Yoga-bhāṣya* explains what is meant by the senses imitating the nature of the mind: "The senses are restrained, like the mind, when the mind is restrained" [YBh 2.54]. Although the *Yoga-sūtras* treat *pratyāhāra* in *Sādhana-pāda*, the chapter on practice, *pratyāhāra* shares with the *antarāṅgas* (the three 'internal limbs' of Yoga-meditation: *dhyāna*, *dhāraṇa*, and *samādhi*) the characteristic that it arises only when necessary conditions are met, rather than being a practice that one can choose to perform, as one can perform *āsana* and *prāṇāyāma*.

> That which is attempted by *pratyāhāra* may therefore be said to be the destruction of [the mind's] natural tendencies and the intrinsic desire on its part to rush out and attach itself to objects, and thereby to bring it under the control of higher and spiritual faculties. . . . *Pratyāhāra* is not therefore the exercise of merely withdrawing the energies working in the senses and centering them in the mind, but of withdrawing the mind from its tendencies to join the senses, and bring its faculties of feeling and willing under control.[70]

Pratyāhāra consists in the senses ceasing their usual functions of contacting objects of perception and transmitting sensory information to the mind. Instead, the mind is fully involved with its object, such as the performance of *prāṇāyāma*, and the usual link between the mind and senses is severed. *Pratyāhāra,* like the components preceding it, utilizes and sublimates the physical body, specifically, the sensory capacities, to prepare for Yoga's higher stages of meditative consciousness.

Cultivation of Consciousness

The Polarity of Samādhi *and* Vyādhi *(Illness)*

Of the many themes that can be explored regarding yogic meditation and higher consciousness, this study of yogic religious therapeutics emphasizes the polarity of *samādhi* or higher consciousness, and *vyādhi*, illness. *Integration* is a pivotal concept in the opposition of *samādhi* (whose nature is *ekāgratā*, one-pointed concentration) and *vyādhi*, which connotes fragmentation. The word *samādhi* means 'putting together' or integrating. It is formed of the prefix *sam*, 'with' or 'together,' and the verbal root √ *dhā*, 'to put,' 'to give.' *Vyādhi* on the other hand is composed of the same verbal root √ *dhā*, preceded by the prefix *vi*, 'out,' 'asunder.' Thus *vyādhi* literally means 'to put out': to disconcert or fragment. Illness is a dis-integrating hindrance to spiritual progress because it keeps one oriented to the physical body and contradicts the recovery of primordial

Unity, named by Eliade the supreme goal of life in the Indian tradition, and "a dream that has obsessed the human spirit from the beginnings of its history."[71] Yoga seeks to counteract dis-integration, whose forms include physical illness and mental distress, to help bring about states of higher knowing and being. *Samādhi* is the quintessential form of reintegration—the recovery of Unity. The polarity of integrated higher knowledge and states of disability opens perspectives on meanings of well-being, both psychophysical and spiritual. *Vyādhi* implies dis-integration or fragmentation. Yoga counteracts dis-integration, which manifests as physical and mental dysfunction and distress.

Yoga's final three limbs or components are called *antarāṅga*, the 'internal limbs' (*antar*, 'inner'; *aṅga*, 'limb'), as distinguished from the first five 'external limbs,' *bahirāṅga* (*bahis*, 'outer') [YS 3.7]. The internal limbs are progressively pure meditative stages. In Yoga's inner limbs, the mind's activity is confined within increasingly focused spheres: first on a particular object of concentration (*dhāraṇā*), then with unwavering awareness of the object in the state of meditation (*dhyāna*), and finally, in the eight stages of *samādhi*, in increasing meditative absorption. *Dhāraṇā*, *dhyāna*, and *samādhi* are together called *saṃyama*, by which one attains *prajñā*: higher, liberative knowledge [YS 3.4,5].

Sixth Limb: Concentration—Dhāraṇā

Āsana and *prāṇāyāma* are practiced to reduce distractions arising from the body/mind, and *pratyāhāra* consists in elimination of mental distraction from sensory sources. On the foundation of these preliminary components, *dhāraṇā* is a further refinement of consciousness undertaken to confine the mind's activity within particular boundaries.

> *Deśa-bandhaś cittasya dhāraṇā.*
>
> Concentration (*dhāraṇā*) is the confining of the mind to one place [i.e., to an object of meditation].
>
> YS 3.1

The word *dhāraṇa* is also derived from the verbal root √ *dhā*, which has meanings including 'to hold,' and refers to holding a chosen object in the mind. Objects that may be chosen for concentration include points in the body, *mantras* or sacred sounds, or an image of a deity or revered master [TV 3.1]. Concentration on an object in *dhāraṇā* is not worship of the object or what it represents; the object merely serves as a single focal point for the mind's complete attention.

Dhāraṇā is an *ekāgratā* a 'fixing on a single point,' but it differs from the *ekāgratā* of *samādhi* states, for in *dhāraṇā*, one-pointedness serves the purpose of comprehension—highly focused, but nevertheless ordinary subject-object comprehension.[72] *Ekāgratā* in the stages of *samādhi*, however, evolves from one-pointed subject-object comprehension to the meditator's absorption in the object of meditation. Yoga's wisdom about human nature is evident in its inclusion of *dhāraṇā*, for *dhāraṇā* provides limited freedom for the mind to consider various aspects of the object of concentration, rather than demanding immediate and complete restriction of the mind's activity. The *sādhaka's* aims in *dhāraṇā* are two: to reduce the frequency of the mind's wandering from the object of concentration, and to increase the magnitude of one's alertness and awareness. Vācaspati notes that *dhāraṇā*, *dhyāna*, and *samādhi* "are related to one another as cause and effect consecutively, and their order of causation is fixed" [TV 3.1]. In Iyengar's *Tree of Yoga, dhāraṇā* is the sap of the tree. As sap pervades all parts of the tree, concentration on a chosen object should pervade the yogin's being.[73] In the present context, where integration is a major factor in healing and liberation, the practice of *dhāraṇā* initiates one-pointedness and provides a bridge from non-fragmented awareness at the level of ordinary cognition, to the fully unified consciousness of *samādhi*.

Seventh Limb: Meditation—Dhyāna

While *dhāraṇā* is the mind's limiting its attention to a single object of concentration, *dhyāna* or meditation is the achievement of sustained and unwavering attention to the object.

> *Tatra pratyayaikatānatā dhyānam.*
> Meditation (*dhyāna*) is the unified flow of the mind in that place [i.e., the 'place' concentrated on in *dhāraṇā*].
> YS 3.2

The transition from *dhāraṇā* to *dhyāna* is spontaneous, not requiring any new technique, and, likewise, *samādhi* is attainable without new techniques once *dhāraṇā* and *dhyāna* are established.[74] While *dhyāna* is the state of full attention to the object of concentration, *samādhi* is the mind's total absorption in it. In Iyengar's model, *dhyāna* is the flower, preceding the fruit of *samādhi*.[75]

The verbal root of the word *dhyāna* is √ *dhi*, 'to think.' *Dhyāna* is not ordinary discursive thinking, but rather the mind's undiluted one-pointed meditation. Progression from *dhāraṇā* to *dhyāna* is represented in the term *pratyaya-eka-tānatā*. *Pratyaya* refers to the effort or contents of the mind, and *eka-tānatā* means "flowing as one" (*eka*, 'one'; √ *tan*, 'to extend,' 'to expand').

> *Dhyāna* may be described as that process by which the mind is constantly concentrated on a single object to the exclusion of other objects in such a way as to put an end to all internal reactions from both past and present impressions, to completely annihilate the very tendency to undergo manifestations and run into all sorts of forms, to overcome all disturbing memories and thoughts, whether pleasurable or painful, and to be able to work with the single impression of restraint, assuming one form and state, and possessing the sole character of the absorbing thought or memory.[76]

The faculty of mental concentration used in Yogic meditation is necessary to all stages of Yoga, and indeed "no profession in this world can we succeed in, if we do not develop this power."[77] However, the concentration exercised in *dhāraṇā*, *dhyāna*, and *samādhi* is a higher form of concentration. Yogic meditation is not of the same order as secular meditation. Eliade is adamant that the experience of Yogic meditation exceeds ordinary meditative experience in purity and density, and, further, that *dhyāna* permits comprehension of the inner form of objects. He gives the example of the meditation on fire, which permits the yogin to have insights such as comprehension of the physiochemical process of combustion, identification of this process with the combustion that occurs in the human body, identification of the fire before him with other forms of fire including the sun, cognizance of fire at the plane of the 'infinitesimals' that compose it, recognition of fire as *prakṛti*, mastery of the 'inner fire' by *prāṇāyāma*, and—by extension from microcosm of self to macrocosm of world—mastery of the actual coals before him.[78]

The passage from *dhyāna* to *samādhi* is marked by the dissolution of distinctions between the subject, object, and process of meditation. Complete integration of experience arises, and the meditator is aware only of "the new ontological dimension represented by the transformation of the 'object' (the world) into 'knowledge-possession.'"[79] This break to a higher order of knowing and being is the yogin's entry into the stages of *samādhi*.

Eighth Limb: Meditative Trance—Samādhi

In *samādhi*, the yogin has consciousness only of the object of meditation, for the mind is 'absorbed' in the object and loses awareness of itself:

> *Tad evārthamātra-nirbhāsaṃ svarūpa-śūnyam iva samādhiḥ.*
>
> Meditative trance or *samādhi* is the same as meditation (*dhyāna*), except that the mind shines with the light of the object alone, and is devoid, so to speak, of its own nature.
>
> YS 3.3

Samādhi is by nature indescribable. It is commonly associated with other-worldliness, but states of consciousness resembling its lower stages are not as distant as one might assume. Iyengar says that *samādhi* is glimpsed by a musician engrossed in playing music, or an inventor making a discovery in a state of concentration devoid of egoism.[80] However, while the first stages of *samādhi* involve ordinary (albeit 'absorbed') cognition, the higher stages require prolonged effort, and constitute a 'raptus' (or rupture of plane), characterized by Eliade as "a passage from being to knowing" leading finally to the fusion of all "modalities of being."[81] The term *samādhi* is translated as 'absorption' or 'trance' (from the Latin *transīre*, 'to go across'). 'Trance' denotes states of consciousness in which one is detached from awareness of sensory stimuli.[82] *Samādhi* is a form of trance, but not all trance is *samādhi*. Hypnotic trance falls in the category of *vikṣipta:* states of mind that are distracted but occasionally steady.[83] *Vikṣipta* is one of the five states of mind listed in the *Yoga-bhāṣya:*

1. Wandering
2. Forgetful
3. Alternately steady and distracted
4. One-pointed
5. Restrained

YBh 1.1

Hypnotic trance is merely a provisional state of concentration, but the trance state of *samādhi* is a sustained one-pointedness. Trance state is characteristic of shamanic practice. However, while shamanic trance is ecstatic—a journeying outside oneself to other regions of the cosmos—"Yoga pursues enstasis, final concentration of the spirit and 'escape' from the cosmos."[84]

The *bhāṣya* on the *Yoga-sūtra's* first verse says that Yoga is *samādhi*. After listing the five stages of mind, the commentator says:

> That however, which in the one-pointed mind, fully shows forth an object existing as such in its most perfect form, removes the afflictions, loosens the bonds of karma and thus inclines it toward restraint, is said

The Eight Stages of Samādhi

SABĪJA SAMĀDHI

(Samādhi 'with seed')

Samādhi with *saṃskāras* (impressions of experience)
productive of mental activity.
Samprajñāta samādhi (= *samāpatti:* coalescence of mind with object)
= cognitive *samādhi*, with support (with object of meditation):
four types of samāpatti (coalescence of mind with object):
Samprajñāta-vitarka: with reasoning (*tarka*) =
cognition of gross elements (*mahābhūtas*) of object of meditation:

1. SAVITARKA SAMĀPATTI: Concentration on gross form of meditation-object with awareness of its name and associated concepts.

2. NIRVITARKA SAMĀPATTI: Concentration on gross form of meditation-object without awareness of its name and associated concepts.

Samprajñāta-vicāra: With discriminative reflection (*vicāra)*=
cognition of subtle elements (*tanmātras*) of object of meditation.

3. SAVICARA SAMĀPATTI:
With awareness of the subtle elements' qualities.

4. NIRVICARA SAMĀPATTI:
Without awareness of the subtle elements' qualities.

5. SAMPRAJÑĀTA-ĀNANDA:
Cognition of intelligence (*buddhi*)
and experience only of bliss (*ānanda*) and ego (*asmitā*).

6. SAMPRAJÑĀTA-ASMITĀ:
Cognition of materiality (*prakṛti*) pure of modification,
and experience only of ego (*asmitā*).

. . . .

Oscillating between stages of *samprajñāta*,
and between *sabīja* (6) and *nirbīja* (8):

7. ASAMPRAJÑĀTA OR NIRODHA SAMĀDHI:
Supracognitive *samādhi*; without support
(without object of meditation).

8. NIRBĪJA SAMĀDHI
Samādhi 'without seed': 'Dharma-cloud *samādhi*.'

> to be the Cognitive Trance (*samprajñāta samādhi*). . . . When however all the modifications come under restraint, the trance is Supra-Cognitive (*asamprajñāta samādhi*)
>
> YBh 1.1

The literal meaning of *samādhi* is 'putting together' (*sam*: 'with'; √ *dhā* 'to put'). Non-yogic meanings of *samādhi* include 'to join,' 'to arrange,' and 'to put in order.' Absorption is a central connotation of *samādhi*: *Samādhiyante asmin iti samādhiḥ*: "*Samādhi* is that in which all is absorbed."[85] Dasgupta renders *samādhi* as "unifying concentration."[86] Connections between *samādhi* and integration include:

1. *Samādhi's* basis: The psychophysical integration that makes *samādhi* possible
2. *Samādhi's* process: Integration of mind with object
3. *Samādhi's* purpose: Reintegration of the yogin with *puruṣa*

Samādhi culminates Yoga's eight limbs, but is not itself the culmination of Yoga. *Samādhi* denotes a range of states of higher consciousness necessary for liberation. Similar to the way the external limbs of Yoga (1–5) are instrumental to the internal limbs (6–8), the lower stages of *samādhi* are instrumental to the higher stages [YS 3.7–8]. The lower stage of *samādhi* is *sabīja*, 'with seed,' that is, with viable *saṃskāras*, literally, 'impressions,' subtle forms of experience, which remain in the mind and produce mental activity and bondage. In *sabīja samādhi*, new *saṃskāras* are prevented, and existing ones are "kept under control and made invisible to the vivifiying impulses from the outside."[87] In *nirbīja samādhi* all *saṃskāras* are destroyed, even the *saṃskāras* generated in *sabīja samādhi* [YBh 1.51]. *Sabīja samādhi* has two varieties: *samprajñāta*, involving cognition applied to objects of meditation (thus called *samādhi* with support), and *asamprajñāta samādhi*, which is supracognitive and without a supporting object of meditation. Eliade writes that in *samprajñāta samādhi* the yogin

> . . . is still conscious of the difference between his own completely purified consciousness and the Self; that is, he is conscious of the difference between *citta* reduced to its luminous mode of being (*sattva*) and *puruṣa*. When this difference disappears, the subject attains *asamprajñāta samādhi*, now every *vṛtti* is eliminated, 'burned'; nothing remains but the unconscious impression (*saṃskāra*) and at a certain moment even these imperceptible *saṃskāras* are consumed, whereupon true stasis 'without seed' (*nirbīja samādhi*) ensues.[88]

The four types of *samprajñāta samādhi* (also called *samāpattis* or 'coalescences' of mind with the object of meditation) correspond to the four states of the *guṇas:* the particular, the universal, the differentiated, and the undifferentiated [YS 2.19], as shown in the table below.

Asamprajñāta samādhi may arise between the stages of *samprajñāta samādhi.* It oscillates between the final stage of *sabīja samādhi* and the dawning of *nirbīja samādhi. Asamprajñāta samādhi* is the *nirodha* stage of *samādhi*, wherein there is no mental activity.

> The mind in this state is in pure vacuity so to say; there are only some of the germs of thought in the form of potencies. The 'I' of the mind remains long in this *nirodha* in a state of absolute objectlessness; all the potencies are destroyed, and at last the *citta* is annihilated in the sense that it returns back to *prakṛti*, never again to bind *puruṣa.*[89]

Nirodha means stoppage (√ *rudh*, 'to stop,' 'to obstruct'). The *nirodha* state is the necessary condition for passage into *nirbīja samādhi*, which involves three 'transformations' or *parināmas: samādhi, nirodha*, and *ekāgratā.* Transformation to *samādhi* is the cessation of 'many-pointedness' and the arising of one-pointedness, *ekāgratā.* This first

The Four Stages of Samprajñāta Samādhi *(The* Samāpattis*)*[90]

VITARKA	*Viśeṣa* or particular *guṇa*-state. *Viśeṣa* refers to the state of the lower mind that regards objects as distinct from one another and separate from divine consciousness.
VICARA	*Aviśeṣa* or universal *guṇa*-state. *Aviśeṣa* designates the higher mind's power to identify universal categories and principles underlying particulars.
ANANDA	*Liṅga* or differentiated *guṇa*-state. *Liṅga* means a mark that identifies. In the *ānanda* or bliss stage, all objects are experienced as part of universal consciousness, yet each remains distinguishable.
ASMITA	*Aliṅga* or undifferentiated *guṇa*-state. *Aliṅga* means without mark or differentiating characteristic. In the *asmitā* stage (awareness of 'I am,' but without bliss), objects lack distinct identity for the yogin. Consciousness is pure: distinct objects of course continue to exist, but the yogin is aware instead only of the whole of *puruṣa.*

transformation is *samādhi parināma*. Then follows *ekāgratā parināma*, where arising and subsiding cognitions are the same. In the third transformation, *nirodha parināma*, the *citta-vṛttis* or 'mind-waves' are suppressed between the arising and cessation of impressions [YS 3.9–12].

With *nirodha* established, and having thus entered *nirbjīa samādhi*, the yogin attains the highest *samādhi: dharma-megha-samādhi. Megham* means 'cloud,' and *dharma-megha-samādhi* is sometimes translated as 'cloud of virtue,' suggesting the pouring forth of rains of goodness, but this is a figurative interpretation. Vācaspati explains *dharma-megha-samādhi* as "the stage when all other thoughts cease to exist, then he becomes possessed of constant discriminative knowledge" [TV 4.29]. Based on Vācaspati's clarification, we might take *dharma* in its meaning of 'thing or object' and surmise that the *dharma-cloud* refers to a state wherein external stimuli and internal saṃskāric impulses are nullified for the yogin, and pure consciousness is experienced, similar to the way things become invisible in thick fog. From the higher knowledge or *prajñā* attained in *dharma-megha-samādhi*, the yogin realizes the distinction of *puruṣa* from *prakṛti*, and is thence liberated, *kevali*.[91] A *jīvanmukta*, one 'liberated in life' has enlightened understanding of his own consciousness as part of the all-embracing *puruṣa*.

The claim that liberation is healing in Yoga is supported by the polarity of *vyādhi*, illness, and *samādhi*, conceived in terms of its integrative qualities. *Vyādhi*, the disintegrative condition of illness, is the first and foremost of the nine obstacles to the integrated state of *samādhi* [YS 1.30]. The word yoga in its sense of 'yoking' itself signifies integration: *samādhi*—whose nature and means of attainment is integration—is the fruit of Yoga practice and the means to liberation. Yoga seeks to counteract psychophysical disintegration, a basic form of which is ill-health. More significantly, Yoga seeks to remedy the dis-integrated state of the mind, so the yogin becomes reintegrated with the primordial power of consciousness that is her true Self-nature.

A number of determinants of psychophysical health are thematic in yogic religious liberation. For example, a chief determinant of health, freedom from pain, warrants the interpretation that the overcoming of suffering resulting from the *kleśas*—afflictions affecting the soul as well as body/mind—is part of attainment of health in an ultimate, spiritual sense. Self-identity is another determinant of health in its ordinary meaning, and is also integral to yogic liberation. By naming establishment in Self-nature as Yoga's aim [YS 1.3], the *Yoga-sūtras* at their very outset ground the claim that Yoga permits the realization of health in an ultimate sense. The concept of integration funds the distinction between *samādhi* and *vyādhi*. In this chapter's final section, "Liberation as Healing in Classical Yoga," conclusions about the therapeutic elements of Yoga's soteriology are informed by analysis of a web of concepts presented to demonstrate the following:

- Commonalities of holiness and wholeness
- The role of integration as a corollary of wholeness
- Freedom and identity as goals of both religion and medicine

LIBERATION AS HEALING IN CLASSICAL YOGA

In classical Yoga, liberation is healing in an ultimate sense. With few exceptions, the Hindu traditions hold that the human body is different from the true Self that is eligible for liberation. The person's fundamental nature is understood as spiritual, rather than physical, psychological, rational, or otherwise, and the Hindu traditions offer religious prescriptions for attaining well-being at the most fundamental level, the spiritual. The term 'health' in its ordinary meaning pertains to physical and psychological well-being, but integral to the claim that liberation is healing is the premise that the extension of the word 'health' can be legitimately broadened to apply to the well-being of the person's ultimate nature.

Healing and Yoga's Therapeutic Paradigm

Analysis of Yoga reveals two major domains of the relationship between health and religiousness:

1. *Health as an aid to religious progress:* purification and conditioning of the body and mind in order to support greater spiritual awareness and progress.
2. *Liberation as healing:* attainment of freedom from limitations and suffering, resulting from realization of one's true Self-nature as consciousness.

According to Vyāsa's *Yoga-bhāṣya*, Yoga and medical science have a common therapeutic paradigm, as shown on the next page. Vyāsa's therapeutic paradigm conveys the fundamental meaning of health in Yoga: ultimate well-being consisting in freedom from limitations and suffering, and, foundational to this, the unimpaired manifestation of Self-identity. A

Yoga's Therapeutic Paradigm in the Yoga-bhāṣya

Medical Science	Yoga
1. Illness	Cycle of suffering and rebirth (*saṃsāra*)
2. Cause of illness	Cause of *saṃsāra:* ignorance (*avidyā*)
3. Goal: Restoration of health	Liberation (*mokṣa):* independence (*kaivalya)*
4. Remedy	Discriminative knowledge (*vivekakhyāti*)

YBh 2.15

therapeutic paradigm can be excavated as follows from these central passages of the *Yoga-sūtras:*

> *Pariṇāma-tāpa-saṃskāra-duḥkhair guṇa-vṛtti-virodhāc ca duḥkham eva sarvaṃ vivekinaḥ.*
>
> All is suffering to discriminating persons, because of misery resulting from change, anxiety, and their subliminal impressions (*saṃskāras*), and because of conflict between the mind's modifications (*vṛttis*) and the basic constituents of matter (*guṇas*).
>
> YS 2:15

> *Heyaṃ duḥkham anāgatam.*
>
> Suffering not yet come can be eliminated (*heyam*).
>
> YS 2:16

> *Draṣṭṛ-dṛśyayoḥ saṃyogo heya-hetuḥ.*
>
> The cause (*hetu)* of suffering is the conjunction of Seer and seen.
>
> YS 2:17

> *Tasya hetur avidyā.*
>
> The cause [of the conjunction of Seer and seen] is ignorance [i.e., *puruṣa's* ignorance of its true nature as consciousness].
>
> YS 2:24

> *Tad-abhāvāt saṃyogābhāvo hānaṃ tad dṛśeḥ kaivalyam.*
>
> By removal (*hanam*) of ignorance, the conjuction between Seer and seen is eliminated, and this is the liberation of the knower.
>
> YS 2:25

> *Viveka-khyātir aviplavā hānopāyaḥ.*
>
> The means of removal (*hānopāya*) [of ignorance] is unwavering discriminative knowing.
>
> YS 2:26

Yogāṅgānuṣṭhānād aśuddhi-kṣaye jñāna-dīptir ā viveka-khyāteḥ.

By practice of the components of Yoga, which destroy impurity, higher knowing shines forth, reaching up to discriminative knowing.

YS 2:28

Yama-niyamāsana-prāṇāyāma-pratyāhāra-dhāraṇā-dhyāna-samādhayo' ṣṭāvaṅgāni.

Yoga's eight components are: moral self-restraints, moral observances, posture, regulation of breath, withdrawal of the senses, concentration, meditation, and meditative trance.

YS 2:29

In an analysis of the four-fold division of the *Yoga-śāstra*, the Āyurvedic medical science, and the Buddha's Four Noble Truths, A. Wezler discusses the term *ārogya*, 'health' (*a* 'not,' *rogya* 'broken,' from √ *ruj*, 'to break'). Wezler notes that *ārogya* connotes *restoration* to a condition free of disease, presupposing an original state of health.[92] In this vein, Halbfass suggests that an important bridge between medical and soteriological 'health' in the Indian traditions is:

> . . . an appeal to the idea of a "return" in a non-temporal sense, a rediscovery and retrieval of an identity and an inherent, underlying perfection that has always been there, and that has to be freed from obscuration, confusion, and disturbance.[93]

His analysis of Sanskrit terms for health indicates that self-identity is central to a concept of health that bridges medical theory and soteriology. *Svāsthya*, 'abiding in oneself' connotes:

> . . . "coinciding with oneself," being in one's true, natural state, free from obstruction; it is a state of health and balance as well as of identity and true self-understanding, "being oneself" in a physical as well as a cognitive sense.[94]

Halbfass observes that in the Indian conception of liberation, metaphysics ultimately transcends medicine,[95] and that the 'health' that Yoga offers "transcends all merely physical healing."[96] This interpretation accords with the view of healing expressed in the *Sāṃkhya-kārikā*, the text providing much of Yoga's metaphysical foundation. Medicine does not relieve suffering with certainty and finality, "therefore, one should entertain a desire for knowledge of those means, other than these evident means, which finally and completely remove misery" (SKB 1.1).

Yoga's Therapeutic Paradigm in the Yoga-sūtras

Heya	To be eliminated: The ailment to be eliminated: *duḥkha*: suffering.	YS 2.15, 2:16
Hetu	Cause of the ailment: The cause of the ailment is misidentification of Self. (knower) and non-Self (knowable).	YS 2:17, 2:24
Hāna	Removal of the ailment: Knowledge of appropriate remedy.	YS 2.25
Hānopaya	Means of elimination of the ailment: Therapy, remedy, medication.	YS 2:26, 2:28, 2:29

Yoga's four-part therapeutic paradigm not only identifies the common healing functions of Yoga and medical science, but also conveys that Yoga offers health of a superior kind. The meanings connoted by the term 'health' depend on our metaphysical conception of the human being. Yoga regards the person's true nature as consciousness, while the body, senses, and mind are considered evolutes of primordial matter, *prakṛti*, the ground of entanglement in materiality, ignorance, and suffering. In Yoga, the true Self as consciousness takes priority over the psychophysical self in establishing the meaning of health. We ordinarily speak of health in reference to the well-being of the body and mind, but at its basic conceptual level, health means wholeness and well-being. Determinants or criteria of physical health derivable from the texts of Āyurvedic medicine are applicable to Yogic liberation—notably, wholeness, integration, identity, and freedom. These Āyurvedic determinants of health are integral to grounding the claim that in classical Yoga, liberation is healing in an ultimate sense.

Wholeness and Holiness

Wholeness in the context of human health connotes a state without impairment and suffering. A holistic perspective recognizes the interdependence of factors constituting person and environment, and that influence states of health and illness. Yoga's prescription for liberation is paradigmatic of holistic treatment of the dimensions of the person. Practice of the eight components of Yoga cultivates human physicality, psychology, morality, and spirituality by integrating the functions within and among these domains. An example is *prāṇāyāma*, control of subtle vital energy achieved by regulating the gross physical action of the breath, which is practiced to help establish the conditions necessary for meditative consciousness. Etymological analysis of both English and Sanskrit terms corroborates the claim that health and holiness have common ground. The modern English word 'holy' descends from the Indo-European root √ *kailo-*, whole. A descendent of *kailo* is the Old English *hāl*, meaning 'whole.' 'Holy' and 'health' are both derived from *hāl.*[97] The word 'salvation,' derived from the Latin *salus*, meaning both 'healthy' and 'whole,' also suggests the idea of healing from the afflictions of the human condition.[98]

The contrast of *vyādhi* and *samādhi*, divergent in respect of integration, invokes Yoga's meaning of yoking, that is, unifying and integrating. Integration is a concept derivative of the concept of wholeness: to integrate is to make something whole by bringing its parts into functional relation. A primary form of integration in Yoga refers to a state of consciousness integrated in the respect that it manifests pure awareness, silent and still, without the awareness-fragmenting distractions of the *vṛttis*, or 'turnings' of mental activity. The first five components of Yoga can help one achieve brief instants of this non-fragmented and integrated concentration in Yoga's sixth component, *dhāraṇā* or concentration. When the state of concentration is sustained, one is in meditation, *dhyāna*. In *samādhi*, integration of consciousness is complete: the mind's potential activities are wholly integrated in one-pointed meditative 'consciousness of consciousness' [YS 3.3; 3.11–12].

The perspective of 'holism' considers entities and systems as composed of, and functioning within, integrated and mutually influential subsystems, rather than as isolated concatenations of separate parts. What is the sense of 'whole' in the context of the holy? The holy is beyond the limitations of the human state and the mundane world. The related term 'sacred' descends from the Latin verb *sacrāre*, from the Indo-European root √ *sak-*, 'to sanctify'[99] and suggests purification and dedication.[100] 'Sacred' connotes that which is pure. In Yoga, purity is the determinant of the sacred. Yoga endeavors to increase purity in body and mental life, attitude and action. To the extent that these are pure, the Self as consciousness may manifest itself. In medical theory, purity is the conceptual category opposite of pathogenicity. Purity in the sense of physical asepsis is a primary concern of medical science, and in the domain of religion, purity is a criterion for distinguishing between the sacred and the profane.

If we leave aside pathogenicity and hygiene from the concept of impurity, we uncover the underlying principle of impurity as 'matter out of place.' This approach, according to Mary Douglas, "implies two conditions: a set of ordered relations and a contravention of that order."[101] In classical Yoga, the order that impurity contravenes is the proper relation of *puruṣa* and *prakṛti*. *Puruṣa* should have contact with *prakṛti* only to the extent necessary for the discrimination of itself from matter. Purity then, means non-attachment to materiality. *Puruṣa* is eternally calm, clear, and at peace, whereas *prakṛti* is unconsciousness, ever agitated and in tension. Entanglement in materiality is impurity. That which is sacred is pure, in virtue of being undefiled by materiality and ignorance. Purity in Yoga, in the most elemental terms, is realization of the primordial wholeness of the spiritual Self.

Identity and Freedom

Medical health and spiritual health both entail freedom from limitations and suffering, and the manifestation of one's identity. Among Sanskrit's etymological reflections of the common meanings of healing and religious liberation is the verbal root √ *muc*, 'to free,' the root of the word *mokṣa*, ultimate liberation. *Muc* can also be used in the sense of healing: *vyādheḥ muc* means to free a person from illness, and from accompanying limitations and distress.[102]

Freedom in Yoga entails liberation *from* the human condition with its inevitable limitations and suffering, but, moreover, liberation *to* the realization of one's true identity. Freedom in the physical domain has both internal and external dimensions. Physical freedom in an outward sense signifies absence of interference to a person's exercise of choice and action. Health is the inward dimension of physical freedom: health is contingent in part on one's vitality and inner resources to accomplish his or her purposes. Actualized self-identity in the context of psychophysical health means having the aspects of oneself functioning together so that their integrity is preserved and one can act in ways that support thriving and accomplishing one's goals. Illness, on the other hand, entails interference with physical and/or psychological functioning, and produces symptoms causing temporary or permanent limitations in the functioning of body and/or mind.

Liberation in Yoga is realization of Self-identity. Although attainment of liberation in Yoga results in well-being and non-suffering, Yoga's ultimate goal is realization of a Self-identity that permits freedom from attachment to objects of pleasure and pain. Non-attachment in turn results in non-suffering. Well-being and non-suffering are merely benefits of liberation, similar to the way that physical health is a valuable result of the physical self-cultivation undertaken to support meditative practice and attainment of liberative knowledge. The ultimate meaning of healing in Yoga is the attainment of identity and freedom; relief of suffering is corollary to this attainment. Relief of suffering and the promoting of well-being are essential attributes of both religion and medicine, and our understanding and practice of medicine and the healing arts can be informed by metaphysical insights gained from *Yoga-śāstra*. An implication for medicine is that healing, like liberation, involves more than relieving impairment and suffering; it means promoting wholeness, integration, identity, and freedom.

In Yoga, health in the psychophysical domain is subsidiary to the wholeness and well-being that is the Self's abiding in its true nature. This follows from Yoga's standpoint on the preeminence of *puruṣa* over *prakṛti*. The inherent wholeness and recovery of well-being of Self is of ultimate value. The body is not only impermanent, but even the greatest physical vitality is irrelevant once attachment to materialist views and experiences is dissolved. Therefore in Yoga, the fundamental meaning of health is the well-being of liberated consciousness, a state wherein wholeness, integration, Self-identity, and freedom obtain, and one attains immunity to the vicissitudes of the material natural world and those of one's own body and mind.

While medical healing is concerned primarily with the particular ailments of individual persons, the idea of religious health invokes well-being that transcends the personal. Progress on the yogic path entails increasingly greater well-being, first at the psychophysical level, then spiritually, as the psychophysical dimension serves its liberative purpose and is transcended. Ultimate well-being is freedom from all that obscures one's spiritual Self. The Self does not require healing, for it is intrinsically whole and well, and not subject to sickness and suffering. Healing in an ultimate sense means curing psychophysical limitations, and limited understandings, that interfere with the recovery of the spiritual Self.

Chapter Four

TANTRA AND AESTHETIC THERAPEUTICS

The various yogas give different priority to the role of the body. Haṭha Yoga, part of the Tāntric tradition, is the form of yoga that most strongly emphasizes physical health and the soteriological role of the body. But even in Haṭha Yoga, the body is a vehicle for the attainment of spiritual aims. The currents of *prāṇa* or vital energy are directed by means of physical disciplines such as *āsana* and *prāṇāyāma*, but the yogin controls these currents of vital energy for the sake of religious realization. The Haṭha text *Gheraṇḍa Saṃhitā* opens with a verse praising Haṭha Yoga as the first rung on the ladder to Rāja or classical Yoga. Eliade observes that the Haṭha texts' repeated assurances that their physical practices "destroy old age and death . . . illustrate the real meaning and final orientation of these techniques."[1] Specifically, liberation and not physical health is Haṭha yoga's ultimate goal.

Classical Yoga assumes the existence of two primordial kinds of being: materiality and consciousness. Yoga does not reconcile this metaphysical dualism by argumentation. Instead, a pragmatic justification is offered for the conjunction and ultimate separation of consciousness and materiality. Metaphysical dualism is integral to classical Yoga's soteriology. Materiality—comprising mind/body and world—is necessary for the Self's experiencing itself and realizing that Self is not of the nature of matter. While Self-realization entails dualism—independence of consciousness from material and psychological nature—at the same time, practice of classical Yoga is paradigmatic of mind/body holism. Yoga's pragmatic holism, however, does not solve the ontological split between materiality and consciousness. Classical Yoga disvalues material nature, the body, relationality, sexuality, and the feminine (which is the gender of *prakṛti* or materiality). These elements are central in the Tāntric tradition, whose monistic ontology is not subject to the problems of metaphysical dualism. Tantra offers alternatives to the ascetic life recommended by classical Yoga. Tantra shares classical Yoga's aim of spiritual Self-realization, but in Tantra, embodiedness and sacredness remain compatible. This chapter treats somatic and therapeutic elements of Tāntric yogas. Tantra adds to the model of religious therapeutics the domain of *aesthetic therapeutics*, that is, healing of body/mind and spirit through sensory experience and religious arts, such as music and dance. As an example of comparative inquiry into religio-aesthetic therapeutics, I explore the healing functions of sacred music.

BODY AND TĀNTRIC YOGAS

Features of Tāntric Practice

Tāntrikas believe that the various religious texts were provided for different eras. The *Kulārṇava Tantra* says:

> For the first of the four world ages *śruti* (Veda) was given; for the second, *smṛti* (the teaching of the sages, *dharmaśāstra*, etc.), for the third, *purāṇa* (the epics, etc.), and for the fourth, *āgama* (the Tantras).[2]

In the *Māhānirvāṇa Tantra*, Pārvatī describes the first *yuga* or age, the *Kṛtya* or *Satya Yuga*, as an age of virtue and happiness. In the second or *Dvāpara Yuga*, *dharma* was disordered and the Vedic rites no longer effective. The third or *Treta Yuga* was marked by the loss of one-half of *dharma*, and illness of people's bodies and minds. The present age is the *Kāli* age: *dharma* is destroyed, and people are gluttonous, malicious, stupid, shameless, and suffering. For this crude age, Tantra is prescribed [MNT 1:20–52]. *The Kāmākhyā Tantra* classifies persons according to three dispositions: the *paśu* or animal, the *vīra* or heroic, and the *divya* or divine.[3] These correspond generally to Sāṃkhya's three *guṇas*: *tamas* (inertia), *rajas* (activity), and *sattva* (awareness). While *sattva* is the ideal in classical Sāṃkhya-Yoga, Tantra holds the *vīra* to be the disposition most suited to the present *Kali* age [MNT 1:54–61]. Tāntric *sādhana* can be undertaken only under the direction of a qualified *guru*, a spiritually awakened person, who grants "an influx of spiritual energy" (*śaktipāta*) which releases potentials from within the aspirant.[4] Some knowledge must be imparted by a *gūru* and cannot be gained from texts. M. P. Pandit writes: "No text gives the *sādhana* in full for it cannot. The crucial part, the *life* of the *sādhana* in fact, is communicated in person, in secret, by the Teacher to the disciple."[5]

Tāntric practice is not restricted to the performance of specific spiritual disciplines, but it is meant to be integrated in all moments of life. Characteristic of the Tāntric approach to daily life is spontaneity and acute attunement with one's environment. Kakar quotes a contemporary *Tāntrika*, a Bengali economist in his early forties, whose family has practiced Tantra for three generations:

> The true tāntrik is always in a state of nonsuppression and enjoyment. The purpose of every moment of life is to experience *ānanda*. *Ānanda* is true enjoyment of everything that comes your way. If there is a heat wave, I will not try to make it less by using a fan or an air conditioner. Nor will I try to put up with the heat by turning my mind away and bearing it in the manner of the Stoics. The true tāntrik puts himself, or rather *is*, in a body-mind state where he *enjoys* the heat . . . as he will enjoy the cold. Ideally, a tāntrik is in such a state of attunement with his environment, with what is possible, that his desire awakens just at the moment that the universe is willing to grant it . . . he has developed his capacity for attention and is intensely aware of where he is and what he is doing at every single moment of time. . . . In fact, in his state of nonsuppression and attunement, a real tāntrik becomes aware a little earlier that others when a storm is due or a heat wave is coming so as to be prepared to enjoy them.[6]

A central principle of Tāntric philosophy is *kriyā*, the principle of spontaneous activity. *Kriyā* has resonance with the Taoist idea of *hsiao-yao yu*, 'free and easy wandering,' or *tzu-jan*: 'spontaneity,' and Sufism's *mauja*, 'free and joyous activity.' Within Hinduism, *kriyā* is comparable to the Vedanta doctrine of *līlā*, the sportive play of *Brahman* by which the universe is created. *Kriyā* is the *sādhaka's* free action, issuing from desirelessness. It is distinct from volitional or ethical action—where will is exerted—and also distinct from neurotic behavior, unfree because it is driven by inner psychological tensions.[7] As regards systematic practice, Tantra's fundamental method, like that of classical Yoga, is meditation. A point of divergence is that while classical Yoga aims for meditative states increasingly free of materiality, in Tantra, symbols are central as supports for meditation. Main forms of Tāntric meditative symbols are *mantras* or sacred sounds, *yantras* or visual symbols, and *mudrās* or ritual gestures. These symbols consolidate and organize energy between practitioner and cosmos. Transformation of energy, *śakti*, is an inescapable fact of existence, and Tāntric *sādhana* uses systematic practices to yoke cosmic energy and manifest it in more sublime ways. Foundational to this is purification, explained by Woodroffe in terms of making the pure *guṇa* called *sattva* (purity and illumination) predominate by utilizing the *guṇa rajas*, the dynamic principle of the two other *guṇas*.[8] Classical Yoga, on the other hand, recommends sattvic or pure activities, foods, and so on, for supporting the predomination of purity.

The aim of Tāntric *sādhana* is reintegration of the consciousness (which is fragmented by various mental activities) and recovery of one's identity with cosmic consciousness, *Param Śiva*. Eliade identifies two stages of Tāntric *sādhana*: cosmicization of the human being, and transcendence of the cosmos. The preeminent sign of transcendence is the *kuṇḍalinī's* union with *Śiva* in the *sahasrāra cakra*.[9] Yogic disciplines of *dhāraṇā* and *dhyāna,* concentration and meditation, are necessary for the interiorization of iconography, a universe of symbols that the *sādhaka* enters and assimilates, incorporating into himself the sacred force sustaining them. The Tāntric approach to *sādhana* is illuminated by *nyāsa*, a practice related to iconographic meditation. *Nyāsa* (√ *nyās*, 'to place') is 'ritual projection' of divinities into various parts of the body:

> The disciple 'projects' the divinities, at the same time touching various areas of his body; in other words, he homologizes his body with the Tāntric pantheon, in order to awaken the sacred forces asleep in the flesh itself.[10]

Pragna R. Shah explains the significance of *nyāsa* as the *sādhaka's* realizing that his body and mind are of the nature of consciousness, and by spreading the presence of consciousness throughout himself, he grasps his primordial divinity.[11] *Yantra* and *mantra* are important tools of Tāntric practice, serving as supports for meditative concentration. More than this, they are emanations of the primordial unity; they embody the cosmic manifestation. In the concrete forms of visual-patterns (*yantra*) and sound-patterns (*mantra*), they are assimilable by the *sādhaka* for the restoration of his own identity with *Param Síva*. A *yantra* is a diagram "drawn or engraved on metal, wood, skin, stone, paper, or simply traced on the ground or a wall."[12] The features of a *yantra* symbolize the elements of creation, human faculties, obstacles to progress, the various breaths, deities, and many other aspects of Tāntric soteriology.

Śrī Yantra contains a series of contiguous triangles, the upward ones representing the masculine *Śiva* and the downward ones the feminine

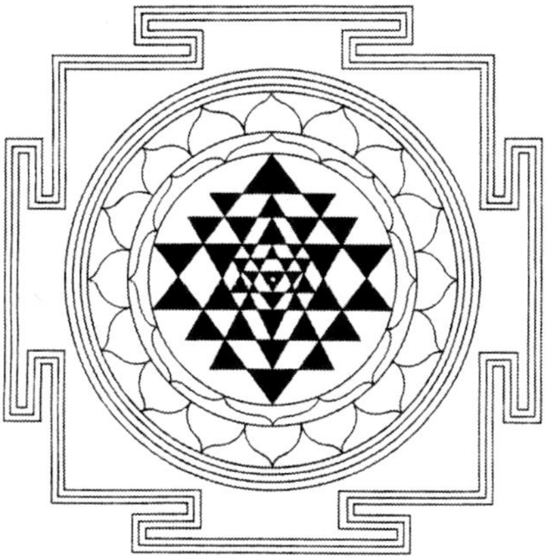

Figure 4.1 *Śrī Yantra*, drawn by John Thomas Casey

Śakti, converging to a central point (*bindu*), signifying the undifferentiated *Brahman*.[13] *Yantra* literally means instrument, or a device to hold or control; its verbal root is √ *yam*, 'to control.' The idea of the *yantra* illuminates the nature of Tāntric practice wherein mystical communication is established with some level of the universe's countless levels, "in order finally to reduce them to unity and master them."[14] John Thomas Casey, who rendered the *yantra* in Figure 4.1, observes that *Śrī Yantra* is naturally captivating to the sense of vision. Concentration on the *yantra* sustains a dynamic tension between archetypal elements such as bounded/boundless, and diversity/unity, evoked by the containing square and the expanding circle. *Śrī Yantra* stimulates multi-planed awareness; a prominent example is the primordial sense of directionality. The four gateways recall the front/back/left/right orientation that conditions the experience of embodied beings. Casey captures the essence of *Śrī Yantra's* power in noting the efficacy of the Great *Yantra* as a meditative object for collecting attention to a single point.[15]

Sexuality in Tantra

Kakar identifies in Tantra "a recognition, even a celebration of man's sensuous nature."[16] This remark should not be taken to mean that Tantra advocates sensual and sexual indulgence, but rather that among the Indian traditions, and even among world religious traditions, Tantra distinguishes itself by its reverence for the body and emphasis on the religious role of physicality. Cosmic energy, *śakti*, takes the form of *kuṇḍalinī* energy in the human body, and sexual energy is among its dominant forms. In the physical enjoyment of sex, this energy is directed downward from the *svādhiṣṭhāna cakra*. In Tāntric practice, directing this energy upward through the *cakras* to the highest one, *sahasrāra cakra,* where union of *Śakti* and *Śiva* takes place, is a divinization of human vital energy.[17] A main reason for Tantra's being misunderstood is its use of a symbolic vocabulary incorporating erotic images. Sexual symbolism is employed in Tantra, but references to the divine coition of *Śiva* and *Śakti* pertain to the polar aspects of reality, and are not meant in gross anatomical terms.[18]

Tantra has been maligned for the 'Five *Makāras*' (five things that begin with the letter *m*): ritual use of wine (*madya*), meat (*māṃsa*), fish (*matsya*), *mudrā* (parched or fried grain), and sexual intercourse (*maithuna*). These elements are not necessary features of Tāntric practice, but, when employed, Tantra requires that they be utilized within the context of worship, without excess, and after purification.[19] As regards ritual sexual union, even among those sects that employ it, some practice it symbolically only. Where ritual sexual union is practiced, its quality is that of Tāntric *sādhana* in general: immobilization. In Tāntric *sādhana's* goal of immobility on the three planes of thought, breath, and sexual sensation, "there is imitation of a divine model—the Buddha, or *Śiva*, pure Spirit, motionless and serene amid the cosmic play."[20] In classical Yoga, the masculine *puruṣa* is the quiescent Seer, and all creative activity issues from the feminine *prakṛti*. Similarly in Tantra, the male aspect is passive, and the female aspect *Śakti* produces all activity. Eliade remarks on Tāntric Yoga's paradoxical arresting of manifestation and disintegration by going 'against the current' (*ujana sādhana*) to recover primordial Unity:

> The paradoxical act takes place on several planes at once: through the union of *Śakti* (= *kuṇḍalinī)* with *Śiva* in the *sahasrāra*, the yogin brings about inversion of the cosmic process, regression to the undiscriminated state of the original Totality; "physiologically," the conjunction sun-moon is represented by the "union" of the *prāṇa* and *apāna*—that is, by a totalization of the breaths; in short, by their arrest; finally, sexual union, through the action of the *vajrolīmudrā* realizes the "return of semen."[21]

Maithuna or ritual intercourse can serve as a support for *prāṇāyāma* and *dhāraṇa* through regulation of respiration and concentration. The goal is the very opposite of sensual enjoyment, and sexual climax is prohibited.[22] Sensuality can be a vehicle that "produces the maximum tension that abolishes normal consciousness and inaugurates the nirvāṇic state, *saṃsāra*, the paradoxical experience of unity."[23] An alternate Tāntric tradition (perhaps the oldest one, according to Banerji) permits sexual climax, "like the offering of sacred oil poured into an altar of fire."[24]

As regards non-ritual sexuality in the context of spiritual life, Mishra indicates that two main qualities are to be cultivated: an attitude of reverence toward sex, and genuine love of one's partner. The *Kulārṇava Tantra* says that the sex act is to be done in the spirit of worship, not for *bhoga* or enjoyment.[25] Sex as given in nature is *bhoga*, but its use as a form of *sādhana* requires its sublimation within a greater spiritual domain. The sanctity of sexuality is warranted in the Indian tradition apart from Tantra. In the *Upaniṣads* one of the manifestations of Brahman 'as food' (i.e., as the outermost sheath of the 'five bodies,' the one supported by food) is the immortality and bliss in the generative organs [Tait. Up. 3:10.2–3]. Other *Upaniṣads* refer to the sexual act in terms of a ritual offering [Bṛhad Up. 6:2.13; Chānd. Up. 5:8.1–2]. In the *Bhagavadgītā* Lord Kṛṣṇa refers to himself as Kandarpa, the deity of desire who empowers procreation [BhG 10:28]. Loving one's partner has the ethical dimension of concern for her or his well-being, and the religious dimension of experiencing primordial unity with that person. The partner makes possible the instantiation of a cosmic polarity wherein non-duality may be realized. Tantra's views of sexuality exemplify the Tāntric leitmotif of using material nature to sublimate that which appears base, and to transform nature so as to reveal its inherent sanctity as part of the sacred body of the Absolute. Mishra writes that sex has become mechanical and insipid in contemporary free-sex society, and that the remedy, from a Tāntric standpoint, is cultivation of love, grounded in religiousness.[26]

Tantra's valuing of the feminine is a characteristic that sets it apart from much of the Hindu tradition. In Tantra's metaphysical foundations, the feminine and the masculine are poles of the *Śiva-Śakti* unity, and in practice women are eligible both to receive and to confer initiation into a religious order. The *Yoginī Tantra*, and the contemporary text *Tantratattva*, highly recommend initiation by a female guru.[27] The Tāntric guru of Śri Ramakṛṣṇa was a woman, Yogeshwari. Despite its commitment to the polarity and cooperation of the masculine and the feminine, Kakar notes that Tantra's texts proceed from the viewpoint of male practitioners, and he suggests that Tantra has "greater resonance for the male psyche and physiology."[28] Other sources indicate that in practice males dominate in Tāntric religious practice and leadership, though the *Śakta* groups actually extend full privileges to females.[29]

KUṆḌALINĪ YOGA

Yoga's universality shines beautifully in its many forms throughout countless Indian schools and sects, Hindu and non-Hindu, Vedic and Tāntric. The incorporation of yoga-practices in a range of Indian religious traditions, and yoga's thriving in the world beyond India, attest to the broad applicability of its methods. There is no pure Veda-based yoga nor pure Tantra-based yoga. Though Patañjali's classical Yoga is one of the six *āstika* or Veda-accepting *darśanas*, it contains elements of Tāntric yoga, a main characteristic of which is the cosmic physiology of the *cakras* ('wheels') and *nadīs* ('rivers'). These are, respectively, the centers and channels of energy in the psychophysical organism. Although classical Yoga sees the body in terms of Sāṃkhya's five elements and Āyurveda's three *dhātus* or supports, the texts of classical Yoga also contain references to the subtle physiology central in Tantra. For example, in the *Tattva-vaiśāradī* Vācaspati discusses meditation on 'the lotus of the heart' between the chest and abdomen, and refers to the *suṣumṇā*, the main energy-channel leading to the highest *cakra* [TV 1.36]. The *Yoga-sūtras'* mystical aspect is evident in Section 3, *Vibhūti-pāda*, the section on extraordinary powers. An example is knowledge of the systems of the body attainable by *saṃyama*, meditative concentration, on the navel-*cakra* [YS 3.30].

Tantra incorporates and adapts the various yogas of the Yoga Upaniṣads, which preceded Patañjali's *Yoga-sūtras*. The approximately twenty Yoga Upaniṣads present a range of yoga practices, including the classical elements of moral restraints and commitments, postures, *prāṇāyāma*, sense-withdrawal, and meditation leading to *samādhi*. But unlike classical Yoga, the Yoga Upaniṣads emphasize the subtle physiology of *cakras* and *nadīs*. The Yoga Upaniṣads in general assume *Brahman* as the one real, and take yoga's goal to be the realization of *Brahman*.[30] Dasgupta finds that Tāntric and other modes of worship were influenced by the Yoga Upaniṣads, and that some yoga practices were developed in accordance with Tāntric Śaiva and Śakta doctrines.[31]

Tantra maintains that there can be cooperation rather than opposition between enjoyment in the world (*bhukti*) and the way of liberation (*mukti*): "Tantra is a meeting ground of *bhoga* (enjoyment) and *yoga*."[32] While classical Yoga aims to 'burn up' the *saṃskāras* or seed-potentials of action, Tantra's approach is the maturation (*paripāka*) of seed-desires by exhausting them through their fruition. Mishra criticizes classical Yoga's concept of 'burning' the *saṃskāras*. While actual seeds can be burnt, Mishra says, the analogy breaks down when applied to human desires. Human desires are part of the Lord's sportive creation of the world, *līlā,* and their actualization into worldly activity is an aspect of the fulfillment of the Lord's creation.[33] Like classical Yoga, Tantra holds that attachment and aversion, not worldly objects themselves, produce bondage and suffering. The Tāntric solution is neither indulgence nor eradication of desire, but enjoyment without attachment. Tantra advises against repression of inclinations, recommending that one *witness* one's thoughts and desires, and not suppress them, thus granting the mind opportunity to sublimate thoughts and desires by integrating them, rather than eradicating them.[34]

The aim of Tāntric yoga is the realization of *Param Śiva*. Fundamental to Tāntric *sādhana* is Kuṇḍalinī Yoga, a form of Laya Yoga.[35] Laya Yoga incorporates the system of the *cakras* and *kuṇḍalinī* energy.[36] *Laya,* from the verbal root √ *lī*, 'to dissolve,' means the yoga of dissolution, that is, the dissolution of self into *Brahman*. Dissolution is explainable in terms of the Sāṃkhya elements:

> In the Tāntric form of Laya Yoga or in *ṣaṭcakrabheda*, the five gross constitutional elements (*pañca mahābhūta*) of both body and universe dissolve in their source. It means during the process of yoga, the earth element dissolves into water, water into fire, fire into air, and air into *ākāśa* (space). And this *ākāśa* element further dissolves into their essence like sound, touch, form, taste, and smell which merge again into intelligence (*buddhi*), egoism (*ahaṃkār*), etc., and ultimately into the spirit or consciousness.[37]

Dissolution into Brahman is sought by means of yogic practices that permit union within oneself of *Śiva-Śakti. Kuṇḍalinī,* from the word *kuṇḍala*, 'coil,' refers to the energy or *śakti* of the universe in the form it takes within the human organism. *Śakti* as *kuṇḍalinī* is conceived as a small snake coiled at the base of the spinal column. Activating and directing this cosmic energy within oneself is at the root of Tantra and of Kuṇḍalinī Yoga. Kuṇḍalinī Yoga may be called the yoga of energy. Its concern is stimulating the ascent of one's vital cosmic energy so that the *kuṇḍalinī* that is *Para-Śakti* may pierce through the several energy-centers or *cakras* (literally, 'wheels'), and unite with *Śiva*, who resides in the highest *cakra*, at and above the top of the head.[38]

> The devī who is *Śuddha-sattvā* pierces the three *liṅgas* [within the *cakras*], and having reached all the lotuses [*cakras*] which are known as *Brahmānadī* lotuses, shines therein in the fullness of her luster. Thereafter in her

> subtle state, lustrous like lightning and fine like the lotus fibre, she goes to the flame-like *Śiva*, the Supreme bliss and, of a sudden, produces the bliss of liberation.
>
> SCN 51

Based on Sāṃkhya's metaphysical scheme of the five basic elements that constitute the cosmos and the human organism, Tantra holds that the *cakras* are subtle essences or *tanmātras* of these elements existing within functional loci of the body. The *Ṣaṭ-cakra-nirūpaṇa* describes the six *cakras* with their associated colors, deities, seed-sounds (*bīja-mantras*) and other characteristics, as shown in the table below.[39]

The *nadīs* or channels that carry the body's energy are 72,000 in number according to Tantra. The most important of them is the *suṣumnā*, which is parallel with the spinal column and leads to the highest *cakra*. The two other main *nadīs* are the *iḍā* to *suṣumnā's* right, and the *piṅgalā* to its left [SCN,1]. The ascent of *kuṇḍalinī* is stimulated by yogic practices such as *āsana* or postures, *kumbhaka* or retention of breath, and *bandhas* or 'locks' (√ *bandh*, 'to bind'). When the *bandhas*

The Seven Cakras

	Cakra	Location	Element	Seed-sound
1	*Mūlādhāra* "Root," "Substratum"	between anus and genitals	Earth	*laṃ*
2	*Svādhiṣṭhāna* "Abode of the self"	at root of genitals	Water	*vaṃ*
3	*Maṇipūra* "Jewel of the navel"	solar plexus	Fire	*raṃ*
4	*Anāhata* "Unstruck" (referring to the unstruck sound)	heart	Air	*yaṃ*
5	*Viśuddha* "Pure"	throat	Space	*haṃ*
6	*Ājñā* "Commander," "one who knows	between eyes	*Mahat* (*Mahat* is the Great: includes all elements)	*Aum*
	Additional to the six, because it is partly within body, and partly beyond it:			
7	*Sahasrāra* "Thousand-spoked"	top of and above head		*visarga* (a release of breath)

are applied to a particular region of the body, such as the *mūlādhāra* or 'root' *cakra*, that region is contracted to concentrate energy there. A related practice is performance of *mudrās* or ritual gestures, which permit manipulation of cosmic energy within the body. Woodroffe explains that these practices "rouse *kuṇḍalinī* so that the *prāṇa* withdrawn from *iḍā* and *piṅgalā* may by the power of its *śakti*, after entry into the *suṣumnā*, or void (*śūnya*) go up to the *Brahma-randhra* (the opening of the *suṣumṇā-nadī* at the crown of the head)."[40] The commentary of the *Ṣaṭ-cakra-nirūpaṇa* provides some sense of how this occurs:

> The yogin should sit in proper posture . . . and steady his mind by the *khecharī mudra*. He should next fill the interior of his body with air and hold it in with *kumbhaka*, and contract the heart. By doing so the escape of upward breath is stopped . . . he should contract the anus and stop the downward air . . . by so doing the fire of *kāma-vāyu* there is kindled, and the *kuṇḍalinī* gets heated (excited) thereby.
>
> SCN I commentary

The text describes *kuṇḍalinī's* ascent and piercing of the *cakras*. Finally she "drinks the excellent nectar issuing from *Param Śiva*." She then returns to her place in the *mūlādhāra* or root *cakra*: "As she returns she infuses *rasa* (the 'juice' of life) into the various things she had previously absorbed into herself when going upward" [SCN 53 & commentary]. *Samādhi* in Tantra is this mystical union of *Śiva* and *Śakti*. Kuṇḍalinī Yoga's conception of *samādhi* is very different from that of classical Yoga, because on the Tāntric interpretation, rather than achieving independence for the body as classical Yoga intends, the body itself participates in enlightenment and liberation. One of the ways body participates in Tāntric practice is in the use of *mantra*, the experiencing of sacred sound.

Mantra Yoga

The idea of mystical sounds has roots in the *Vedas*. The great seed-sound *Aum (Om)* is the source of, and the summation of, all sounds.[41] *Aum* is identified in the *Yajur-veda* with *Brahman*, with the *Vedas*, and with eminent gods. In classical Yoga, *Om* is the designator of the Lord Īśvara. The *Brāhmāṇas* contain *mantras* later used in Tantra, but it remained for Buddhist and Śaiva Tantra to accord *mantra* the status of a vehicle of salvation, *mantrayāna*.[42] Speech is the mother of creation in the Hindu tradition. In the *Ṛgveda*, *vāc*, the personification of speech, says:

> I bring forth the Father, at the summit of this (cosmos). My womb (origin) is within the waters, in the ocean. Thence I extend myself throughout all the worlds; yonder heaven also I touch with my peak.
>
> I also blow forth (pervading everything) like the wind, taking to myself all the worlds. Beyond the heaven, beyond this earth, so have I become in grandeur.
>
> RV 10: 125.7–8 (trans. Edgerton)

Mantra Yoga uses the ontological power of the word in the context of Tāntric *sādhana's* interiorization of cosmic forces. A *mantra* is a 'seed-sound' or sequence of seed-sounds, called *bījas* (*bīja*, 'seed'). Each *mantra* has "a characteristic pronunciation and intonation that the disciple normally learns from his *gūru*."[43] The verbal root of *mantra* is √ *man*, 'to think,' but more broadly, 'to consider,' 'to learn,' 'to understand.' As regards the meaning of *mantras*, some are composed of actual words, while others are composed purely of non-word combinations of seed-sounds. In either case, the seed-sounds comprising the *mantra* have esoteric meanings understood by the *mantra's* possessor. *Mantras* transcend the realm of representational language; the seed-sounds are considered to be of the nature of *Brahman* and manifestations of *Śakti* or cosmic energy. According to the *Viṣva-sāra Tantra*, *Brahman* in its fundamental form as sound, *śabda-brahman*, is the substance of all *mantras*, and exists in the body of the person, *jīvātma*. *Śabda-brahman* has an 'unlettered form' *(dhvani)*, that is, a primal sound not produced by the human voice, and also a 'lettered' form (*varṇa*), which is produced by the voice. *Dhvani* is the source of *varṇa*, and is a subtle aspect of the *jīvā's* vital *śakti*.[44] *Mantra* is a 'symbol' in the archaic sense: "It is simultaneously the symbolized 'reality' and the symbolizing 'sign.'"[45]

Important practical and philosophical aspects of mantra are the use of the *bījas* or phonemes as supports for concentration and "the elaboration of a gnostic system and an interiorized liturgy through revalorization of the archaic traditions concerning 'mystical sound.'"[46] A central instance of the interiorization of mystical sound is Kuṇḍalinī Yoga's concept that each of the *cakras* has a certain number of petals on which appear the written forms of particular seed-sounds or *bīja-mantras*, together comprising the forty-nine sounds of the Sanskrit alphabet.[47] Consonant with the Vedic view that the world emerged ultimately from the vibration of *śabda-brahman*, the sounds of the Sanskrit alphabet are thought to embody the constituent energies of the universe, and thus the sounds are sometimes called *mātṛkā* 'sources' (*matṛ*, 'mother').[48] In Woodroffe's words: "as from a mother comes birth, so from *mātṛkā* or sound, the world proceeds."[49] L. P. Singh writes that each letter of *mātṛkā varṇa* is living energy: "They are the acoustic root of the different waves and vibrations of the cosmos. These letters are the representative sonoric manifestations of the universe."[50]

A *bīja-mantra* is a mystic symbol ending with a nasal sound, written in Sanskrit's Devanāgarī script with the sign called *anusvāra:* a dot above the syllable. The *anusvāra* is transliterated by an *m* with a dot either above or beneath it: ṁ/ṃ. Sometimes an alternate symbol is used: the *anunāsika*, which means 'through the nose. The *anunāsika* is also called *candrabindu*, 'dot within a moon': (ँ). The sound indicated by these signs is pronounced somewhat like the *-ng-* in the English word fi*n*ger, or so*ng*. When intoning *bīja-mantras*, the nasal ending is not pronounced as an *m* sound, at the lips, but is "sounded nasally, high up in the bridge of the nose."[51] This is why *mantras* written in Roman transliteration sometimes end with *-ng* instead of *m*. Basically, a *bījā-mantra* consists of a single nasalized seed-sound, but compounds such as *Hṛīm* and *Aiṃ* are also called *bījas*.

Bīja-mantras serve as supports for meditation, and as the *sādhaka* progresses, their sounds, and their written forms on specific petals of the *cakras*, are said to become perceptible by mystical or supra-empirical hearing and vision. *Om* or *Aum* is written ॐ, with stylistic variations. *Aum* is the seed-sound of the sixth *cakra*, in the region between the eyes, and its ending is a labial *m* sound. *Omkāra*, the primordial sound *Om*, is said to be heard spontaneously when the *kuṇḍalinī* rises and opens the 'inner vision' of this 'third eye.'[52] The location of the *bīja-mantras* at the various *cakras* is not arbitrary, but expresses a precise physiocosmic correspondence: The fifty primordial sounds (the forty-nine + *kṣam)* have points of resonance within particular regions of the body. For a simple demonstration, chant the fourth *cakra's* seed-sound *yaṃ*, and the *bīja*-petal sounds *kaṃ, khaṃ, gaṃ, ghaṃ*, and so on. Compare the vibration in the area of the fourth *cakra*, the heart region, against the locus of vibration of *haṃ*, the seed-sound of the fifth *cakra* in the throat region (its *bīja*-petal sounds begin with vowels: *aṃ āṃ, iṃ īṃ,* and so on).

Mantra's efficacy depends in part on the fact that, correctly recited, *mantras* can 'become' what they represent:

> Each god, for example, and each degree of sanctity have a *bīja-mantra*, a "mystical sound" which is their "seed," their "support"—that is, their very *being*. By repeating this *bīja-mantra* in accordance with the rules, the practitioner appropriates its ontological essence, concretely and directly assimilates the god, the state of sanctity, etc.[53]

The *Mahānirvāṇa Tantra* gives instructions for use of the mantra *Om Saccidekaṃ Brahma:* "O, the One-Being-Consciousness Brahman" [MNT 3:12–49]. A sense of how the *bīja*-sounds embody both meaning and ontological power is conveyed in the text's unfolding of *Om* (*Aum*) to reveal that *A* signifies the protector of the world, *U* its dissolver, and *M* its creator [MNT 3:32]. Eliade notes that a whole system of metaphysics may be concentrated in a *mantra*, citing the Mahāyāna Buddhist text *Aṣṭasāhaśrika-prajñā-pāramitā*, progressively reduced to the *mantra* '*pra*,' by which practitioners are supposed to grasp the meaning of *prajñā-pāramitā* metaphysics.[54]

There are three main forms of *mantra* recitation: *vācanic* or aloud, *upanṣu* or silently with the lips moving, and *mānasika* or mental. While Vedic hymns are chanted aloud, Tantra considers silent *mantra*-recitation superior.[55] The repetition of *mantra* is called *japa. Mantra-japa* has the power, according to Bhartṛhari's *Vākyapadīya*,[56] to remove ignorance, reveal truth, and lead to realization of liberation. *Mantras* may also be used in preparation for activities of daily life, making the practitioner receptive for an awaiting experience.

For instance, a *mantra* composed of the sounds *Vaṃ*, *Aiṃ*, and *Aiṃ-Vaṃ* is recommended in preparation for listening to music. The *bīja Aiṃ* represents the goddess *Sarasvatī*, deity of language, music, and learning.[57] According to Kakar, *Aiṃ* is associated with the state of wonder, while *Vaṃ* is a sound used as an opening syllable when the practitioner is aiming for a state of expanded awareness.[58] Such a *mantra* is considered purificatory:

> . . . this clears the practitioner's inner ear, and prepares his mind to enjoy the music . . . used in this way, the *mantra* acts as a ritual which raises the emotional level of the user to a point where the actual signals are received with the utmost clarity and acted on in the most appropriate way.[59]

In the *Yoga-sūtras*, where spiritual progress depends on the stilling of the *vṛttis* or turbulent activities of the mind, *mantra* is recommended for stilling the mind by meditation on God. Classical Yoga's second limb, *niyama*, includes *svādhyāya*, study, and one kind of study is repetition of *Om*, the designator of Īśvara [YBh 2:32].

> The mind of the yogin who constantly repeats the *praṇava* (*Om*) and habituates the mind to the constant manifestation of the idea it carries (i.e., Īśvara), becomes one-pointed.
>
> YBh 1:28

The commentary invokes the Vedic assertion of the coexistence and eternal relation of a word and its meaning, and implies that knowledge arising from the mantra *Om* leads ultimately to direct perception of Īśvara.[60] In *Ṣaṭ-cakra-nirūpaṇa*, however, a fundamental application of *mantra* is the rousing of the dormant *kuṇḍalinī* by the *mantra Hūṃ-kāra* [SCN 50]. Liberation according to both classical Yoga and Tantra requires freeing the mind of its fragmentive activity. *Mantra* is a yogic practice that is therapeutic in virtue of its power to counter the dissipation of mental energy, and to channel the *sādhaka's* power to realize a higher state of being.

AESTHETIC THERAPEUTICS IN TANTRA

Hinduism's therapeutic impetus is evident in Śaṅkara's speaking of ultimate liberation as health, *svāsthya,* 'self-abiding,' and all the way back to this hymn to Rudra (Śiva) in the *Ṛgveda*, among the most ancient texts on earth:

> May I attain a hundred winters, O Rudra,
> through the most comforting remedies given by you!
> Drive away from us enmity, farther away distress,
> away diseases—in all directions!
> . . . Bring us across to the further shore of distress
> for our well-being. Keep away all onsets of infirmity!
>
> . . . Cause our heroes to thrive with your remedies!
> I hear of you as the best physician of physicians.
> RV 2:33.2–4 (trans. Maurer)

If it is granted that liberation is healing, in the sense of gaining freedom from limitations and suffering, each of the many Hindu religious and philosophical traditions can be seen, on its own terms, as having some therapeutic concern. In seeking a more comprehensive account of religious therapeutics, the initial model derived from classical Yoga and Āyurveda is next expanded with Tantra's 'aesthetic' therapeutics. I understand *aesthetic* not only in reference to art, but also in its original sense, pertaining to sense perception [Gk. *aisthenasthai*, 'to perceive'].[61] Tantra's concept of the body as part of the sacred creation, and as an instrument and subject of enlightenment, opens the way for aesthetic forms of religious practice, such as music and dance, whose therapeutic properties are both psychophysical and spiritual.

Therapeutic Elements of Tantra

Tantra's impetus as a religious therapeutic is evident in the *Mahānirvāṇa Tantra* when Śakti addresses Śiva as "Lord among physicians of earthly ills" [MNT 4:7]. The word used for ills is *bhavavyādhi*, explained by Woodroffe as meaning "both the ill of existence itself (i.e., the cycle of rebirth and death), and the ills flowing therefrom."[62] Among Indian traditions, Tantra is outstanding for its concern with practical problems over philosophical ones, and on this basis, Basu notes Tantra's affinity with the art of medicine.[63] Eliade locates the source of Tantra's therapeutic concern in its conception that the great ailment of human life is 'suffering.' Suffering, in soteriological terms, arises from "the shattering of the primordial Unity," co-extensive with the creation and coming-to-be of all things.[64] Tāntric religious therapeutics therefore focus on the recovery of unity, particularly utilizing somatic experience for meditation and attainment of liberative knowledge. Psychologically, Tantra implies that the healthy personality is integrated—not fragmented—especially in virtue of its recommending that desires be sublimated or otherwise recast, rather than being eliminated or repressed. Kakar puts it this way:

> The healthy personality in Tantra is neither passive nor desireless; it has only redefined the terms of the struggle between desire and a world which is often unable and unwilling to gratify it.[65]

Tantra, with other Indian traditions, promotes liberation by means of knowledge, but (like classical Yoga), its psychophysical therapeutics are liberative as well.[66] Tantra holds that ignorance of the identity of self and ultimate reality produces spiritual illness, and perpetuation of the cycle of death and rebirth. Shah identifies a range of therapeutic applications of Tāntric theory and practice, presenting perspectives on health conceived in terms of equilibrium among Yoga's five *prāṇas* or vital airs, Āyurveda's three *doṣas*, and the five *mahābhūtas* or basic elements of Sāṃkhya.

Shah examines the therapeutic powers of four manifestations of *kuṇḍalinī* energy. Its *kriyavatī* aspect is *kuṇḍalinī's* manifestation on the physical plane. This is the domain of vital energy resulting from practice of Haṭha Yoga. *Kuṇḍalinī's kalavatī* aspect pertains to energy manifest as the digestive fire, whose function is necessary for physical health. The *vedhamayī* aspect concerns the rising of *kuṇḍalinī* through the *cakras*. Each *cakra* is associated with a particular *mahābhūta* or element, and with cultivation of one's power to control the ascent of *kuṇḍalinī*, the *sādhaka* is said to be able to influence the five elements, whose proper proportions determine one's state of health. Finally, the *varṇamayī* aspect concerns pronunciation of the *varṇas*, the sounds of the Sanskrit alphabet. Each of the forty-nine sounds is a manifestation of the *vaikhari* or audible form of *śabdabrahman*, and according to the Tāntric text *Śarada Tilaka*, each sound is associated with either the *iḍā-nadī* (governing vital currents), or the *piṅgala-nadī* (governing mental currents). For instance, short vowels are contained in *piṅgalā* and long vowels in *iḍā*. To appreciate how this functions concretely, pronounce aloud and compare the different qualities of the Sanskrit short vowel *a* ('uh'), and the long vowel *ā* ('aah'). Shah hypothesizes that the excess of *vital* current can produce erratic functions within the body-mind complex, while the excess of *mental* current may lead to physical inflexibility and rigidity in the personality.[67]

Vyaas Houston, founder of the American Sanskrit Institute (Warwick, New York), corroborates the claim that oral Sanskrit can influence psychophysical states. In his discussion of how a person can become exquisitely aware of the unique resonance of each of Sanskrit's forty-nine sounds, he compares the effects of uttering aspirated and unaspirated consonants:

> . . . one of the great pleasures of the Sanskrit language lies in the alternation between minimal-breath and maximal-breath consonants. The minimizing of breath while producing a consonant, when for example, touching the tip of the tongue behind the teeth in *ta*, brings about an intensely focused one-pointedness of concentration; while a consonant released with maximal breath, like *tha* has an expansive liberating effect. It releases pressure from the heart and chest, and creates a happy relaxed feeling.[68]

Māntric utterances thus have application as a religious therapeutic using the medium of speech: correct pronunciation of suitable combinations of letters produces resonances that can equilibrate the circulation of energies in a person. Shah writes that this therapeutic application of kuṇḍalinī's *varṇamayī* aspect can be performed by a healer on behalf of a patient. The first three aspects, however, can be utilized only by an individual whose Tāntric practice has developed her power to use *kuṇḍalinī's* manifestations on behalf of her own health.[69]

Sacred Music

Tāntric music and dance are religious arts expressing the two fundamental manifestations of primordial *Śakti* or energy: vibration and movement. Śiva is known as *Naṭeśvara*, lord of the dance (√ *naṭ* 'to dance').

This appellation reflects the Tāntric conception of constant motion within the cosmos. A dancer, through ritual gestures (*mudrās*), becomes attuned to, and manifests, the rhythms of the cosmos, thus instantiating (for self and for those witnessing the dance) the primordial oneness of self and *Brahman*. This function of ritual dance is religiously therapeutic: dance serves to restore well-being by permitting direct experience of—and thus knowledge of—the relation of self with the sacred. Religious dance has therapeutic properties in the psychophysical domain as well. For the better expression of mood and meaning, a dancer utilizes the yogic practices of breath control (*prāṇayāma*) and postures (*āsana*) to gain calmness of mind, physical fitness, and flexibility.

Music, too, is a manifestation of the cosmic *Śakti*. The *Nāda-bindupaniṣad*, which instructs about the yogic liberative practice of listening to the 'inner sound', articulates the value of sound for developing meditative concentration:

> The mind, the snake abiding in the hole of the interior of the body, caught by (the snake-charmer of) sweet sound, completely forgetting the world, does not run anywise, becoming one-pointed.[70]

The 'inner sound,' *nāda*, is one of the levels of the manifestation of *śabda-brahman*, or the Absolute as Sound. *Nāda* is supra-sensuous sound, audible only with sufficient meditative effort and purification of the *nadīs* or nerve currents. The *Yoga-śikhopaniṣad* distinguishes four forms of *śabda-brahman*. The most subtle is *para-śabda* or supreme sound, associated with the *mūlādhāra* or root *cakra*. Next is *paśyanti-śabda*, 'visible sound,' by means of which yogins see the universe. It is associated with the *anāhata cakra* of the heart area. *Anāhata* means 'unstruck,' and refers to self-generating sound. *Paśyanti-śabda* is also known as *anāhata*, sound that does not issue from material vibration. The unstruck sound is heard as the *praṇava*, that is, the sacred sound *Om*, which is according to the *Yoga-sūtras*, the designator of Īśvara. The third form of *śabda-brahman* is *madhyama-śabda*, 'middle sound,' designating the forty-nine sounds of the Sanskrit alphabet. Finally, the coarsest form of sound is *vaikhara-śabda*, 'manifest sound,' whose manifestation is speech.[71] Tantra, even with its emphasis on the body, recommends silent recitation of mantra. This attests to the strength of the Indian inclination to transcend or sublimate physicality. Both 'inner' and 'outer' sound are important in Tantra, but in the context of body and religiousness, physically audible sound—particularly in the form of sacred music—is important in Tantra's aesthetic therapeutics.

Rāgas, or melodic frameworks, cultivate meditative awareness in both musicians and listeners. The verbal root of *rāga* is √ *raj* or *rañj*, 'to color' 'to please': "Hence the term occupies a rich semantic field that includes such things as color, feeling, intensity, passion, love, and beauty. The primary aim of a *rāga*, then, is to bring delight by stimulating an emotional response in the hearer."[72] From a Tāntric standpoint, *rāgas* can calm and concentrate the mind, and stimulate it aesthetically in the direction of religious realization.

Whether or not one accepts Tāntric interpretations of how dance and music can contribute to spiritual realization, Tantra provides useful articulations of the spiritual potential of engagement with art. Tantra embraces the somatic and the aesthetic within its religious domain, and provides a conception of art that is both therapeutic and religious. If we take the term *aesthetic* in its fundamental meaning of pertaining to sense experience, and the term *art* in its broader connotation as applicable to forms that evoke meanings beyond themselves, Tantra indicates that the realm of aesthetics can be a significant dimension of religious therapeutics. Insight into religious therapeutics in the domain of aesthetics could be developed by considering the healing applications of religious expressions such as Navajo and Tibetan sand-paintings, and the use of sacred music, dance, and other arts in a range of traditions.

SACRED MUSIC AS A RELIGIOUS THERAPEUTIC

Across world traditions, sacred music is valued for its healing powers, for example, in the peace and well-being induced by hearing Gregorian chant, and the use of indigenous American (American Indian) medicine songs sung in curing ceremonies. The Tāntric conception of body as an instrument of liberation grounds a notion of sacred music as a religious therapeutic, as does the notion of *śabda-brahman*, sound as the origin and fundamental expression of being. The Kashmir Śaiva text *Spandakārikā* (Stanzas on Vibration) conveys that the purpose of *mantra* is the achievement of unobscured consciousness. The following passage from the commentary *Spandavivṛti* of Rājānaka Rāma expresses that the use of mantra for physical healing is of the same order, but of a lesser degree that the use of mantra for the imparting of supraphysical wholeness:

> (Mantras) that have not become one with the supreme Lord [by "seizing the strength" associated with Śiva] are no more than mere phonemic sounds, subject to creation and destruction. . . . However, by laying

> hold of that strength, their powers to perform their functions, be they of a superior order (such as the imparting) of initiation of an inferior, (such as) remedying (the effects) of a scorpion's venom, transcend all limitations.[73]

From the standpoint that liberation is healing in the ultimate sense, the following discussion uses Tāntric foundations to illustrate inquiry into a specific theme—sacred music—showing how music functions as a religious therapeutic. Comparative applications emphasize the healing power of sacred music in a variety of Asian and American Indian traditions. Three main themes are addressed:

- Sound as a focus for meditation and a stimulus to the expansion of liberative knowledge and consequent well-being.
- The healing and liberative efficacy of breath-control in song, chant, and the playing of wind instruments.
- The function of music for experiential identification of Self and the sacred.

Harold Coward writes that in all world religions, the oral experience of scripture is as important, or more important, than the written:

> The dominance of the written text for contemporary Westerners is partly a result of the impact of modern, print-dominated culture on religious experience. But it is quite out of line with the traditional experience of scripture as found in the world religions and in Native American religious experience. In each tradition the scripture began orally and to varying degrees has remained a basically oral phenomenon.[74]

Not only spoken and heard scripture, but other forms of language are important in religious life: performative speech, chant, and song can all be used in a sacred manner. By *sacred* in this context I mean that language and music are ways of experiencing relatedness with what is holy. Both classical Yoga and Tantra incorporate the power of mantra as a focal point for meditation, and a stimulus to the realization of one's true nature and well-being. Vācaspati's commentary on the *Yoga-sūtra* says that repetition and understanding of *Om* is "the means of feeling the presence of the Lord everywhere, in all circumstances and phenomena" [TV 1:28]. Sound is so important in Tāntric practice that Tantra is also called *Mantra-śastra*. Tantra articulates the theme of ritual identification of (forces of) Self with (forces of) cosmos. One of the most palpable ways to experience this identification is in the production and perception of sacred music. The word *sādhana*—devoted practice of a discipline for the purpose of spiritual self-healing and enlightenment—can apply to sacred music.

How Is Sacred Music Therapeutic?

Clearly music can be religious—in its content, and its power to induce reverent and even meditative states. Music also symbolizes (participates in and points to) sacred forces. But how is sacred music therapeutic? A non-dualistic concept of the person, conceived not as a compound of the two substances 'mind' and body'—but described by terms 'mind' and 'body' to designate two main dimensions of human experience—entails a theory of etiology or causation of disease wherein mental and physical states are understood as mutually influential. A fundamental manifestation of this phenomenon is the fact that emotional distress activates neurochemicals that can compromise vitality and immunity. Conversely, mental calm has a healthful effect on the body. Sacred music serves many functions, and one of them is to calm the mind/body so that well-being can prevail. Physician Harold G. Koenig comments on numerous medical studies concerning neurochemical health factors:

> Persons who are depressed have increased secretion of cortisol, from the adrenal glands. This natural substance interferes with the immune system, which is the body's major defense against cancer, infections, and other outside invaders. In fact, this is the substance that doctors give patients who receive heart, kidney, or liver transplants to suppress their immune systems so that their bodies will not reject the transplanted organ. Psychological distress also causes the adrenal glands to secrete epinephrine and nor-epinephrine, substances that cause constriction of blood vessels, which may contribute to high blood pressure, diseases of the arteries that feed the heart (coronary arteries), and possibly irregularities in hearth rhythm (arrhythmia). Finally, psychological stress increases activity in a part of the nervous system called the autonomic nervous system, which may cause or worsen heart and blood vessel problems, as well as induce stomach ulcers, and many lower bowel or colon problems. Consequently, persons with emotional problems such as depression, anxiety, or those who are under chronic stress may be under greater risk of dying from a number of stress-related diseases.[75]

In addition to the physiologically therapeutic benefits of religious experience, including participation in sacred music, a deeper appreciation of sacred music as a religious therapeutic is possible on the interpretation that religious liberation is itself healing. Music's healing effects in the psychophysical dimension contribute to religious realization equivalent to fundamental healing of our human condition.

Breath, Music, and Healing

A fundamental inspiration for inquiry into music as medicine is Yoga's prescription of control of the breath for establishing meditative consciousness. In using the word *inspiration* here, I wish to convey its double meaning of stimulation of feeling or creativity, and its literal meaning, from the Latin *inspirāre* 'to breathe into.' The force behind sacred speech and song is breath. Air is the constant support of our physical life, and breathing is the fundamental human interaction with the energy of the cosmos. The medium of the sound of the flute is breath, the vehicle of *prāṇa,* the current of life. To play the flute requires control of breath, not *prāṇāyāma* as it is practiced for yogic meditation, but with *prāṇāyāma*'s essential property of specially timed inhalation and exhalation, and, more important, its effect: breaking the tendency toward breathing that is thoughtless and erratic. Instead, the breathing is regulated and a meditative state ensues from the quieting of what classical Yoga called the *vṛttis*, the 'turnings' of mental activity. Ordinary breathing tends to be shallow, but in *prāṇāyāma* and other breath-disciplines, breath is made more even, and deeper breathing infuses the body/mind with vitalizing oxygen, in turn infusing the practitioner spiritually with more *prāṇa.*

In Navajo philosophy, the word *niłch'i* is translated by James K. McNeley as 'Holy Wind':

> Suffusing all of nature, Holy Wind gives life, thought, speech, and the power of motion to all living things and serves as the means of communication between all elements of the living world.[76]

Health and well-being are central concerns in the Navajo worldview. The term *hózhó* has meanings along the lines of beauty, harmony, order, and well-being. Through ritual, *hózhó* is restored to an individual's being, and through speech and song, *hózhó* is then imposed into his universe, carried by *niłch'i*:

> After a person has projected *hózhó* into the air through ritual form, he then at the conclusion of the ritual, breathes that *hózhó* back into himself and makes himself part of the order, harmony, and beauty he has projected into the world through the ritual mediums of speech and song.[77]

Pacific Northwest traditional healer and oral historian Johnny Moses (*Whisstemenee:* Walking Medicine Robe) is a member of the Nootka and Tulalip nations, and a practitioner of a medicine way called *SiSíWiss*, which means *Sacred Breath*. He says:

> Singing and sound can change the way you think or how you feel. We use healing songs to strengthen people and to help them discover the richness of their being. We have songs that can even heal a person who is suffering.[78]

Moses explains that the Samish word *sī'īlh* means 'to sing,' 'to pray,' and 'to cry.' In expressing the healing power of sacred song Moses says, "We believe that when you sing, your cry will turn into a song.[79] He says of healing ceremonies: "We sing for a person in sorrow to uplift them, to give them energy, to give them life-force."[80] Breath has special significance here: sacred songs carry the breath of the ancestors, which continues to help and heal the living generations. Not printed words, but the breath-infused words of traditional teachers, healers, singers, and the oral historians known as storytellers perpetuate healing knowledge and the spirit of life.

Body as Instrument of Sacred Music

A major feature of Tantra is the ontological presupposition that the universe, and everything in it, is a manifestation of the one Brahman. Emergent from this principle is a positive attitude toward material nature and the human body. Tāntric practice utilizes material nature in order to transcend subjugation to materiality. Tantra regards the body as part of the sacred creation, and as enlightenable itself. Tāntric religious therapeutics focus on recovery of the primordial unity of Self as cosmos, and utilize somatic experience for meditation and the attainment of liberation. Music is a manifestation of primordial *śakti* or energy. Swami Prajñānānanda explains that the *nāda śakti* or primordial sound energy is experienced by both musician and listeners:

> Gradually the awakened energy penetrates all the force centers of the body and finally reaches the thousand petalled lotus of the *sahasrāra* . . . and then the *sādhaka*-artist and the sincere music listeners feel divine communion of the *jīvātman* and *pāramātma*. They attain the fruition of the *nāda sādhana*, which enables them to cut asunder the knots of nescience and realize the transcendental Brahman.[81]

The human body is the instrument of sacred speech and song. William Powers' study of Lakota sacred language utilizes Levy-Bruhl's idea of 'appurtenances' to explore the idea of speech and song as extensions of the body.[82] Sacred music can be vocal or instrumental. Sacred music played on instruments extends song from the human performer so that it resonates, not in the musician's voice-box, but in an object, such as a drum. Fundamental musical instruments (after the human voice) are the drum, the rattle, and the flute. In the Lakota language the names of these instruments show that musical instruments are conceived as extensions of the body: The drum is *waapapi*, 'things struck with the hands,' the rattle is *wayuȟlaȟlapi*, 'things rattled with the hands,' and the flute is *wayajopi*, 'things played by blowing.'[83] These instruments, made with a array of designs and materials, have religious and therapeutic uses throughout world cultures.

The voice of the drum is the heartbeat of Mother Earth. It is not that the drumbeat *represents* her heartbeat, but the drum makes audible the pulses of nature, of which our heartbeats are an instance. Drumming is a discipline that can bring about a meditative state. It does this by making audible a regular rhythm that is stabilizing to one's heart and other vital rhythms, and to one's mental rhythms as well. Stabilization of psychophysical rhythms, as yoga demonstrates, induces meditative states of consciousness. Drumming or listening to drumming can accomplish this in a very powerful and direct way because the drumbeat is not only heard with the ear, but its vibrations are felt throughout the body. In the social dimension, the drum can have great unifying power for a group of people, be they marching together, dancing, singing, playing music, listening to music, or participating in ceremony.

Breath is the physical force that produces the sound of the flute. Riley Lee is an ethnomusicologist and master of the *shakuhachi*, a Japanese flute traditionally made of bamboo. Asked about the therapeutic value of playing the *shakuhachi*, Lee jests that his family could dispel the myth that this flute-master lives an entirely serene life. Lee observes however, that playing the instrument has the therapeutic benefits of reciprocally requiring and developing relaxation in three areas of the body that are significant energy-centers, and which tend to accumulate tension: the jaws, the diaphragm, and the occipital area where the neck joins the skull. As regards the function of the *shakuhachi* for religious liberation, Lee notes the use of the flute by Zen monks who play it as a bridge to meditative consciousness and liberation, in some cases playing only one song all their lives.[84] Despite Lee's admission that his life can be very hectic, to hear and see him play the *shakuhachi* is to witness the musicianship of a person whose psychophysical integration and vitality allow him to play music whose sound is sublime—uplifting to the spirit—and is thus both therapeutic and religious.

ELEMENTS OF HEALING IN SANSKRIT CHANT

Among forms of sacred speech and song, sublimity is wonderfully manifest in Sanskrit chant. Like music, Sanskrit uplifts the heart. Houston writes:

> Sanskrit is a language designed for maximum uninterrupted resonance. It is language as music, attracting the full attention of the speaker or singer with the articulation of each syllable blending perfectly without the slightest friction into the next syllable.[85]

Sanskrit sounds are combined according to rules of euphonic combination called *saṃdhi* ('union,' from *sam*, 'together,' √ *dhā* 'to put'). *Saṃdhi* permits "the most perfect uninterrupted flow of the most euphonic blending of letters into words and verse." For instance, the greeting *Namaḥ te*, "Salutations to thee," becomes *Namaste;* the sounds are blended to maintain a current of resonance. In the chanting of Sanskrit scripture or of *mantras*, the experience of unbroken resonation pervades one's entire body and extends beyond oneself.[86] To send forth one's voice, and feel its vibration join the vibrations of the world extending all around oneself, can be a direct and marvelous experience of primordial unity. The rules of *saṃdhi* serve purposes of efficiency and aesthetics in both oral and written Sanskrit, but *saṃdhi's* greatest importance is the power it gives Sanskrit as a vehicle for inducing meditative consciousness, and the higher knowledge that meditative consciousness supports. Other features of Sanskrit also serve this purpose. An essential feature of the language is the purity of Sanskrit's basic sounds, described by Houston as "a coherent selection of the most pure, distinct, and focused sounds that can be made by the human vocal instrument."[87]

The breath-patterns required for chanting is another feature of Sanskrit that supports meditative awareness. For instance, the arrangement of the consonants in the Sanskrit alphabet is based in part on alternation of aspirated and unaspirated sounds, such as *ta* and *tha*. According to the *Taittirīya Upaniṣad*, pronunciation requires attention to sound, accent, quantity, force, articulation, and combination [Tait. Up. 1:2]. Correct pronunciation both requires and cultivates breath-control, and thus chant, like the playing of the flute, has qualities like those of *prāṇāyāma:* regulation of breath leads to calming of the *vṛttis*, the activities of mind that produce bondage and suffering. Meditative awareness gained in Sanskrit chant is thus rooted in the physical experience of:

1. Vocal sound-resonation
2. Control of breath
3. One-pointed concentration required to produce the sounds of the *mantra* or verse being chanted.

Acute attention to locating the precise point of articulation of a sound (for instance, *guttural*, in the throat, or *labial*, at the lips), along with attunement to the correct use of breath to produce the sound, counters fragmentation of consciousness and helps one to develop the one-pointedness of mind prescribed by Yoga.

The somatic and aesthetic dimensions of Sanskrit exemplify the soteriological role of the body in the experience of sacred sound. We ordinarily think of language as a cognitive phenomenon, and regard the physical articulation of speech as incidental to the communication of meaning. Certainly language exists to convey meaning, but the meanings in Sanskrit's awesome body of literature are carried by currents of sound with amazing beauty, and the power to modify states of consciousness. Mental concentration on Sanskrit verses, and the resonation of their sound with one's own body as its instrument, can be an experience of the highest order of enjoyment, a therapeutic that utilizes human physicality in a sublime way.

Healing in Identification of Self with Cosmos

Harold Coward explores how the spoken word can "evoke the Divine word of which it is an earthly resonance."

> A direct correspondence is seen as existing between the physical vibrations of the noumenal chant and the noumenal vibrations of the transcendent. The more the physical vibrations of the uttered chant are repeated, the more Transcendent power is evoked in experience until one's consciousness is purified and transformed.[88]

An instance of religiously transformative chant is Tibetan overtone chanting. Individual monks chant not single notes, but multiple-note chords. Coward writes that chanting "enables the monks to feel the evocation of the interdependence of the universe—a meaning that can be said symbolically in the chanted sounds and gestures, but not said explicitly."[89] Tibetan Buddhist overtone chant expresses that things are more than they seem: the higher overtone frequencies are held to stand in the same relation to the extremely low fundamental tone as spiritual reality stands to the world we think we inhabit.[90]

The flute, by means of breath, has the sound of the wind, so its music easily evokes experiencing the unity of self and cosmos. Kevin Locke (Tokeya Inajin), a Lakota musician and instrument maker, says of the flute:

> . . . the flute is the essence of the wind, especially *Niya Awicableze*, the Enlightening Breath, the first waft on which the meadowlarks return to the Northern prairies. The flute gives voice to the beauty of the land and is the sound of the wind as it rustles the grasses and leaves, scales the buttes and mountains, or skims the surface of lakes and streams.
>
> To send forth the clearest sound the flute must be made with great care and understanding of how the wind-like breath of its user will move invisibly through the flute to draw out a beautiful melody. The music becomes the means of a mysterious unseen communication that flows from one heart to another, one spirit to another.[91]

The flute can sing the sound of the wind in a canyon, and the musician is the locus of the canyon-wind's reinstantiation as sound made by human intelligence, breath, and the instrument he has crafted. Flutes are generally made of plant materials, marking another dimension of the relationality of beings realizable through sacred music. The part of a tree used to make a flute is not severed from the living creation. It continues to live, not biologically, but as a resonator for the breath of a human being, and a resonator for the voice of the wind. Locke speaks of the sounds of the four prime instruments as vehicles of the life-force, and as means to experience one's identity with the creation and its sacred forces. The religious and therapeutic power of music is conveyed in Locke's likening the music of these instruments to the thunderstorms that allow the prairies to bloom. The drum is the thunder "that shakes the human heart out of its slough of despondency." Flute songs are "the wind that purifies and breathes life into the human heart." The rattle's sound is the refreshing rain, and the human voice is streaks of lightning that "illuminate the heart and charge it with energy and enlightenment."[92] The power of sacred instrumental music is all the greater if the musician has crafted his own instrument and experiences the unity of creation in his transforming—for example, part of a cedar tree into a flute with a living voice.

Sound as a Bridge Between Substantial and Non-substantial Being

Sound is physical—it involves energy being conducted through air (a material medium of distantly spaced molecules) and impinging physically on the hearer's eardrum, even impinging on the hearer's body. But sound is not 'material' in the sense of substantiality: sound is not a substance extended in space. Experiencing the reality of the non-material realm through experiencing sound is a powerful way to realize the reality of the spiritual, with spiritual connoting, in part, non-materiality. The opposition of the material and the spiritual does not, however, imply the opposition of the material and the sacred, for 'spiritual' and 'sacred' are not equivalent terms. Furthermore, unlike traditions such as Advaita Vedānta and classical Yoga that regard materiality as inferior, Tantra and indigenous American religious philosophies esteem the natural world and human physicality as compatible with the sacred. Traditions such as these ground the idea of music as medicine.

In the Hindu view of language, it is the 'vibrating' spoken word that has power; words are manifestations of the Divine.[93] Chant issues from a material source—the human body/mind. But even though the resonation of the chanting voice is physical, *it is not material*. Thus it provides direct experience of the reality of the spiritual. The singer's voice radiates out from his body/mind into the atmosphere, creating a field of sound that joins with the field of vibration in which all Being participates. Sacred song transforms consciousness in a healing way. In singing, the vibrations of sound return to the singer, and egoism is destroyed with his awareness, not that he is chanting, but that he is an instrument resonating the song of that which is sacred. In this attunement, the singer can be as an unstruck drum, resonating in concert with the musical vibrations surrounding it.

Conclusion

COMMUNITY: RELATIONALITY IN RELIGIOUS THERAPEUTICS

The model of religious therapeutics presented in this study received its basis from classical Yoga (branches 1–5), and was supplemented with Āyurvedic medical therapeutics (6), and Tāntric aesthetic therapeutics (7). Now to complete the model, the domain of *community* is added, using Hindu and other world traditions, to produce the following set of branches.

Branches of Religious Therapeutics

1. Metaphysical and epistemic foundations
2. Soteriology (theory of salvation or liberation)
3. Value theory and ethics
4. Physical practice
5. Cultivation of consciousness
6. Medicine and health-care
7. Aesthetics
8. Community

This study addressed the problem that the psychophysical person is bound to struggle with problems concerning embodiment and health, and took the position that the spiritual Self suffers no illness, thus religiousness offers a means of realizing one's primordial wholeness and freedom. I assumed the Hindu standpoint that healing, in religious terms, does not mean curing the spiritual Self, for the spiritual Self is not subject to sickness. I argued that *healing* in a religious sense means overcoming impediments that interfere with *realizing* (i.e., *knowing* and *achieving)* one's Self-nature in its full identity and freedom. Classical Yoga, which provided a foundation for the model of religious therapeutics, aims for the transcendence of material nature. But even though classical Yoga provides an extensive system of religious therapeutics, it neglects relationality, for its goal is *kaivalya*, 'independence' of Self as consciousness from entanglement in material nature, including the body, nature, and sociality. Having integrated into the model Āyurveda's holistic contribution to the understanding and preservation of health, and Tantra's approach that enlightenment is attainable through physicality and aesthetic experience, the model now requires a component embracing relationality. The idea of *community* embodies meanings of relationality between person and the sacred, among persons, and among the aspects of creation.

The idea of community thus has applications in the domains of religion, human social life, and ecology. In religion, community refers to participation in, or contact with, that which is sacred. The word community derives from the Latin *commūnis*, 'common,' which connotes shared interests. The Indo-European root of *common* and *community* is √ *mei*, 'to change,' 'to go,' 'to move.' Derivatives of the root *mei* refer to the exchange of goods and services. *Mei* and its derivative 'common' also produce the word *communication*, pertaining to the transmission of information or meaning. In the context of religious therapeutics, communication includes prayer, ritual speech, scripture, and sacred music, which are vehicles for communicating with the sacred, and for conveying among human beings various means of getting in contact with the sacred.

Tantra holds material nature as sacred, thus grounding the valuation of relationality, and among Indian traditions, Āyurveda gives the most attention to the significance of the biophysical environment, as illustrated by Āyurveda's view of pharmacology. Pharmacology is a major branch of both Āyurveda and contemporary scientific medicine. The Āyurvedic view of pharmacology exemplifies Āyurveda's ethos of bio-spiritual community. Plants, which provide food and medicine, are central in Hindu religious cosmology. Exploration of community in the context of religious therapeutics spans themes including sacred song, and human beings' relationships with plants. In the spirit of honoring relationality within the many domains of life embraced by religious therapeutics, consider these verses from the *Upaniṣads:*

The essence of things here is the earth.
The essence of the earth is water.
The essence of water is plants.
The essence of plants is a person *(puruṣa)*.
Chānd. Up. 1:1.2

Agni or 'fire,' the transformative energy of the life process, exists not just in the human being but throughout living nature. In the plant kingdom, photosynthesis is one of *agni's* manifestations. The plants we consume as food and medicine transmit *agni* to us. When digestive *agni* is strong, food affords maximal nourishment, but when *agni* is weak, compromised digestion can contribute to disease. Plants in Āyurvedic pharmacology and dietetics have both medical and religious significance:

> Herbs can transmit that *agni* to us, their capacity to digest and transform, and this may augment our own power of digestion, or give us the capacity to digest substances we normally cannot. The *agni* of plants can feed our *agni*. Through this interconnection, we join ourselves with the cosmic *agni*, the creative force of life and healing.[1]

Frawley and Lad invoke this Upaniṣadic view in examining connections between plant medicines and *mantras*. Both regulate *prāṇa:* similar to a *mantra's* transmitting the seed-energies of consciousness into the mind, medicinal plants transmit the seed-energies of nature into the body to restore well-being.

Traditions such as Buddhism, Neo-Confucianism, and indigenous religions of the Americas and other continents show the importance of community—ecological, social, and spiritual. The religious potential of human relationality with nature emerges in David Kalupahana's examination of the Buddhist understanding of freedom or *nirvāṇa* in terms of health or ease (*sukha*). Freedom is attainable by overcoming egoism, so that passion, hatred, and confusion can be eliminated. "Living in surroundings where one can realize the interdependence of human life and nature" can support the gaining of knowledge that destroys egoism.[2] Kalupahana conveys that natural surroundings—the forest grove, the empty abode—provide a retreat from "the attractions and repulsions generated by artificial forms of life." Physical and mental health are better sustained in unpolluted, natural environments, thus early Buddhist *aramas* or monasteries were generally simple residences surrounded by woods or orchards.[3] Beyond nature's supporting human well-being, the natural world itself possesses Buddhahood, according to some Chinese and Japanese

Buddhists. William R. LaFleur investigates the soteriological role of nature according to the twelfth-century Buddhist monk Saigyō, whose use of natural 'images' in his poetry serves to "create a union of the subject and the real object of his image-ing, that is, the Reality itself."[4] Kūkai (eighth/ninth century), founder of Japan's Shingon school of Buddhism, explains the Buddhahood of plants:

> The *Dharmakaya* consists of the Five Great Elements within which space and plants-and-trees [*sōmoku*] are included. Both this space and these plants-and-trees are the *dharmakaya*. Even though with the physical eye one might see the coarse form of plants-and-trees, it is with the subtle eye that the subtle color can be seen. Therefore, without any alteration in what is in itself, trees-and-plants may, unobjectionably, be referred to as [having] Buddha [-nature].[5]

Kūkai posits the identity of the Buddhist Absolute, the *dharmakaya* or 'body of the *dharma*' "with all forms and things in the phenomenal, mundane world."[6] For Kūkai and Saigyō, concrete phenomena in nature have a soteriological function, at once symbolizing and participating in the Absolute.

Plants are one of the four basic elements in Lakota metaphysics as explained by Lakota elder Wallace H. Black Elk. The four elements are fire, water, rock, and green. *Green* refers to the plants that Grandmother Earth grows out of her body. Black Elk describes being in the woods, experiencing the plants breathing and communicating among one another: "I am part of it," he says, "so there's a chemical language. I was happy there knowing I was related to them."[7] Black Elk is conversant with the discourse of Western disciplines, in which he identifies fours 'languages': the scientific, legal, psychological, and religious. Here he uses the word *chemical* to invoke a context of relationality in which living plants exchange life-force with other participants in the web of life.

Ecologically, community pertains to the relations among all the entities that constitute nature. Life and health in biological terms (for the person as 'the body of food' in Hindu terms) depend on the nourishment extracted from other life-forms within the food chain. In human social life, health and healing depend in part on relations with others. In this connection, Kalupahana says that early Buddhism did not seek to "enable a person to attain spiritual health and not be part of this world." The disease of suffering, caused by craving, is not merely an individual, psychological matter; elimination of craving requires reforms at the level of community:

> It involves a complete change in ideology, whether it be in economics, sociology, politics, or morals. It is freedom or *nirvāṇa* not in a world that transcends the world of experience, but one in which the individual and society enjoy the best of health and happiness.[8]

The Buddha identified malnutrition as a disease, and as a cause of the root disease: suffering. Physical malnutrition is a prime threat to health, and was identified by the Buddha as destructive of the moral fabric of society. Thus individuals' having adequate means of earning a living is foundational to the health of individual and society.[9]

Health influences, and is influenced by, community. Health is not just a matter of one's own systems functioning well within oneself; health requires that entities and systems throughout a community participate in mutually helpful exchanges. Besides the fact that health is contingent on community in terms of factors such as food supply, the healing process itself requires community, but *community* conceived more broadly than human social community. To request healing is to appeal to a source outside oneself to help restore well-being. In saying this I do not deny the innate power of self-healing. In fact, healing must ultimately be generated from within oneself, but its instigation may come from a source that somehow redirects or infuses energy to permit the re-establishment of integrity in the affected system.

The request for healing may be made of such sources as a medical practitioner, a religious practitioner, a human community, a deity, or a tradition, such as Yoga. I have argued that identity is an integral determinant of health: Part of what it means to be in health is to have the aspects of oneself functioning in a sufficiently integrated way, so that one can participate in experiences that manifest and sustain one's Self-nature. Against the view of classical Yoga, I submit that identity can be found in relationality. To have knowledge of, and actualization of, one's Self-nature means to establish one's identity in relation to something. The relation may be conceived from the standpoint of the Upaniṣadic statement of the relation of the individual self or *Ātman* with the one Brahman: *Tat tvam asi,* "That thou art." Or the relation may be conceived, as it is in classical Yoga, in the terms "I am not that," by locating one's identity in *puruṣa*, consciousness, and recognizing that one is not of the nature of matter or *prakṛti.* In Tantra, Self-nature is realized in terms of identity with nature and the divine. Lakota religion, as another example, suggests the realization of self-identity in terms of *relatedness* with the natural world and sacred forces. The Lakota invocation *Mitākuye Oyas'iṇ*, "All

My Relations," uttered at the conclusion of prayers and sacred songs, and at completion of stages of ritual, embodies a cosmological, religious, and ethical recognition and reverence for the interdependence and sacredness of all aspects of creation.

Far from being the 'absence of disease,' health is life's natural tendency. Order and well-being are not just prevailing properties of life, they are warp and woof. Nature's tendency is toward thriving—adaptation, equilibrium, and development. In the religious domain, the human being in its true nature is whole and well, needing only the healing that removes impediments to its perfect nature. The fact that health is fundamental is evident in the miraculous fact that, most of the time, we don't get sick, despite the fact that we continually come in contact with infective agents and other threats: physical, biological, and psychological. When we are sick or injured, healing means restoration of original order and well-being. When, for instance, a leg is broken, medical treatment restores that leg, recreates its real nature, reestablishes its identity as *my* leg, and my identity as one who walks.

To request healing is to affirm health as fundamental to our nature. *To recognize that we need healing*, whether for physical or emotional conditions, or in religious terms, for our human limitations and suffering, *presupposes the order and well-being of life*. To heal is to recover primordial unity, the non-fragmented state in which aspects of self are operating in community, and the person participates in community with other beings in the biophysical and social environments, and with the forces of the sacred, however conceived. *Community* designates webs formed of many kinds of participation and interaction among the constituents of life. Human life depends on community, grounded in interaction and communication. The provinces of community encompass the assimilation of oxygen and nourishment, companionship and love between persons, management of institutions for social welfare, and in the domain of religiousness, fulfilling one's relation with that which is sacred.

Health is fundamental to nearly every human enterprise, and is thus an important consideration in planning and evaluating situations in contexts such as social welfare and education. The determinants of health suggested in this study, for instance, *development* and *freedom from pain*, are offered to contribute concepts and vocabulary for supporting well-being in a variety of settings. The themes that emerged in analysis of determinants of health (biological and ecological, medical and psychological, sociocultural and aesthetic, and metaphysical and religious) are echoed in the reconstruction of the model of religious therapeutics. Our various fields of knowledge offer diverse conceptual and methodological resources for understanding and perpetuating health. This study suggests for further inquiry and action related to health, not just inter-disciplinary but *transdisciplinary* approaches. In other words, we can do more than apply concepts and methods of philosophy, medicine, religion, anthropology, and so on, and (after the manner that holistic medicine recommends focusing on the patient and not the science) take the human being, not the discipline, as a starting point. In responding to the wholeness of the human being, we can create more integrated—and thus more healing—constellations of the registers of human knowledge.

Whether the body is conceived as different from the person's true nature, to be transcended along with the rest of material nature, as classical Yoga holds, or whether body is considered part of the sacred creation and integral to religious life, body remains essential to religious communication. Communication can be accomplished by language, both oral and textual, but in a large share of religious communication, the body is indispensable. Sacred language and songs, and practices such as Yoga's *āsana*, *prāṇāyāma*, and meditation techniques are formalized means of contacting the transcendent, of realizing one's sacred Self-nature. The performance of formalized means of religious communication requires the body, and their transmission depends on a living teacher, one who has mastered them, not just cognitively, but who carries the knowledge of their proper use in her or his psychophysical self.

Inquiry into the body in Hinduism reveals not a Cartesian material body, but a range of concepts of body as a conscious locus of activity, a system of subsystems participating in active relation within a web of other systems—biophysical, social, and spiritual. Examples are the *Upaniṣad's* five sheaths model, the *Bhagavadgītā's* 'field' conception of the person, Āyurveda's ecological view of body and land as the two kinds of place, and Tantra's identification of person as a physioconscious microcosm within the physioconscious world macrocosm. Each of these concepts of the human being counters not only the Cartesian view of body, but counters the stereotype that the Indian traditions assume a dualistic view of body and Self.

One's religious aim might be transcendence of the body, or religious realization in one's embodied state, but, in either case, our journey in this world is an embodied one, and religious life demands our reconciling in some way the dimensions of sacredness and physicality. The larger share of humanity is not inclined toward ascetic life; therefore it is valuable to articulate connections between religiousness and healthful living that utilize and support wholesome physicality, and healthful community life. All our activities—in householding, work, relationship, social welfare, recreation, the arts, and so on—can be performed in a spirit that affirms wholeness and holiness.

> *Om!* One should reverence the Udgītha (song) as this
> syllable, for one sings the loud chant beginning with '*Om.*'
>
> The essence of things here is the earth.
> The essence of earth is water.
> The essence of water is plants.
> The essence of plants is a person.
> The essence of a person is speech.
> The essence of speech is the Ṛg (hymn)
> The essence of the Rg is the Sāman (chant).
> The essence of the Sāman is the Udgītha (song)
> The Ṛg is speech.
> The Sāman is breath.
> The Udgītha is this syllable *Om.*[10]
>
> *Om!*—This syllable is the whole world . . .
> . . . *Om* is the Self indeed . . .[11]

Notes

INTRODUCTION: THE IDEA OF RELIGIOUS THERAPEUTICS

1. Paul Tillich, "The Meaning of Health" in *Religion and Medicine, Essays on Meaning, Values, and Health*, ed. David Belgum (Ames: The Iowa State University Press, 1967) 11–12.

2. *Oxford English Dictionary* [*OED*], 2nd edition, 20 volumes. Prepared by J. A. Simpson and E. S. C. Weiner (Oxford: Clarendon Press, 1989) 14:525–26, s. v. 'save'; 16:36, 'soteriology.'

3. *OED*, 14:420, s. v. 'salvation.'

4. *American Heritage Dictionary*, Appendix: "Indo-European Roots" (Boston: Houghton Mifflin, 1981) 1541, s. v. 'sol-.'

5. *OED*, 14:525–26, s. v. 'save.'

6. *OED*, 17:904–05, s. v. 'therapeutic.'

7. Wilhelm Halbfass, *Tradition and Reflection: Explorations in Indian Thought* (Albany: State University of New York Press, 1991) 250.

8. Kenneth Zysk, "Mantra in Āyurveda" in *Understanding Mantras*, ed. Harvey P. Alper (Albany: State University of New York Press, 1989) 134.

9. Vamberto Morais, "The Contribution of Yoga to Modern Life" in *The Nature of Religious Man*, ed. D. B. Fry (London: Octagon Press, 1982) 129.

10. John M. Koller, "Human Embodiment: Indian Perspectives" in *Self as Body in Asian Theory and Practice*, ed. Thomas P. Kasulis, Roger T. Ames, and Wimal Dissanayake (Albany: State University of New York Press, 1993) 46–47.

11. Halbfass, *Tradition and Reflection*, 250.

CHAPTER 1: BODY AND PHILOSOPHIES OF HEALING

1. Plato, *Phaedrus*, 64c-67b. *Collected Dialogues of Plato*, ed. Edith Hamilton and Huntington Cairns (Princeton, NJ: Princeton University Press, 1961).

2. Friedrich Nietzsche, *The Will to Power* [1901], trans. Walter Kaufmann and R. J. Hollingdale (New York: Vintage Books, 1968) 131.

3. Friedrich Nietzsche, *Thus Spake Zarathustra* [1892], trans. R. J. Hollingdale (Baltimore, MD: Penguin Books, 1977) 62.

4. Eliot Deutsch, *Creative Being, The Crafting of Person and World* (Honolulu: University of Hawaii Press, 1992) 59.

5. Roger T. Ames, "The Meaning of Body in Classical Chinese Philosophy," in *Self as Body in Asian Theory and Practice*, ed. Thomas P. Kasulis, Roger T. Ames, and Wimal Dissanayake (Albany: State University of New York Press, 1993) 164. First published in *International Philosophical Quarterly* 24 (1) March 1984.

6. Ames, "The Meaning of Body in Classical Chinese Philosophy," in *Self as Body*, ed. Kasulis et al., 158.

7. Deutsch, *Creative Being*, 62.

8. Maxine Sheets-Johnstone, ed., *Giving the Body Its Due* (Albany: State University of New York Press, 1992) 2.

9. Drew Leder, *The Absent Body* (Chicago and London: University of Chicago Press, 1990) 4.

10. René Descartes, *Discourse on the Method*, in *The Philosophical Writings of Descartes*, 2 vols. Trans. John Cottingham, Robert Stoothoff, and Dugald Murdoch (Cambridge: Cambridge University Press, 1984, 1985) 1:151.

11. Cited in Richard B. Carter, *Descartes' Medical Philosophy: The Organic Solution to the Mind-Body Problem* (Baltimore and London: Johns Hopkins University Press, 1983) 7.

12. Carter, *Descartes' Medical Philosophy*, 8.

13. Carter, *Descartes' Medical Philosophy*, 22.

14. Carter, *Descartes' Medical Philosophy*, 22–24.

15. Descartes, *Description of the Human Body*, in *Philosophical Writings*, 1:134.

16. *Ouvres de Descartes*, ed. Adam and Tannery, Vol. 4:161–170, 345–48, cited in Carter, *Descartes' Medical Philosophy*, 96–97.

17. Albert A. Johnstone, "The Bodily Nature of the Self or what Descartes Should Have Conceded Princess Elizabeth," in *Giving the Body Its Due*, ed. Sheets-Johnstone, 19.

18. Robert Stoothoff, Translator's Preface to *Passions of the Soul*, in *Philosophical Writings of Descartes*, 1: 325.

19. Johnstone, "The Bodily Nature of the Self," in *Giving the Body Its Due*, ed. Sheets-Johnstone, 22.

20. Descartes, *Meditations on First Philosophy*, Second Meditation, in *Philosophical Writings*, 2:17.

21. Maurice Merleau-Ponty, *Phenomenology of Perception*, trans. Colin Smith (London: Routledge and Kegan Paul, 1962).

22. Sheets-Johnstone, "The Materialization of the Body: A History of Western Medicine, A History in Process," in *Giving the Body Its Due*, ed. Sheets-Johnstone, 133.

23. William Heidel, Hippocratic Medicine, 128–29, cited by Sheets-Johnstone in "The Materialization of the Body" in *Giving the Body Its Due*, ed. Sheets-Johnstone, 147.

24. Francis Zimmermann, *The Jungle and the Aroma of Meats: An Ecological Theme in Hindu Medicine* (Berkeley: University of California Press, 1987) 120, 129.

25. David Michael Levin and George F. Solomon, "The Discursive Formation of the Body in the History of Medicine," *Journal of Medicine and Philosophy* 15 (1990) 518, 519.

26. Sheets-Johnstone, "The Materialization of the Body," in *Giving the Body Its Due*, 142.

27. N. H. Keswani, *The Science of Medicine and Physiological Concepts in Ancient and Medieval India* (New Delhi: All India Institute of Medical Sciences, 1974) 25.

28. Sheets-Johnstone, "The Materialization of the Body," in *Giving the Body Its Due*, 134.

29. Levin and Solomon, "The Discursive Formation of the Body," 524.

30. Levin and Solomon, "The Discursive Formation of the Body," 528.

31. Levin and Solomon, "The Discursive Formation of the Body," 530.

32. Levin and Solomon, "The Discursive Formation of the Body," 533.

33. Wilhelm Halbfass, *Tradition and Reflection: Explorations in Indian Thought* (Albany: State University of New York Press, 1991) 265.

34. Halbfass, *Tradition and Reflection*, 237.

35. Halbfass, *Tradition and Reflection*, 275.

36. John M. Koller, "Human Embodiment: Indian Perspectives," in *Self as Body*, ed. Kasulis et al., 45.

37. Koller, "Human Embodiment," in *Self as Body*, ed. Kasulis et al., 47.

38. Koller, "Human Embodiment," in *Self as Body*, ed. Kasulis et al., 48.

39. Fritz Staal, "Indian Bodies," in *Self as Body*, ed. Kasulis et al., 59–60.

40. *Tattvārtha-sūtra* 5.16, cited in Staal, "Indian Bodies," in *Self as Body*, ed. Kasulis et al., 60.

41. Koller, "Human Embodiment," in *Self as Body*, ed. Kasulis et al., 47–48.

42. Halbfass, *Tradition and Reflection*, 269–73.

43. Koller, "Human Embodiment," in *Self as Body*, 46.

44. Wimal Dissanayake, Introduction to Part Two, "The Body in Indian Theory and Practice," in *Self as Body*, 41–42.

45. Diane B. Obenchain, "Spiritual Quests of Twentieth-Century Women: A Theory of Self-Discovery and a Japanese Case Study," in *Self as Person in Asian Theory and Practice*, ed. Roger T. Ames, Thomas P. Kasulis, and Wimal Dissanayake (Albany: State University of New York Press, 1993) 127.

46. S. C. Banerji, *A Brief History of Tantra Literature* (Calcutta: Naya Prokash, 1988) 1–5.

47. Surendranath Dasgupta, *A History of Indian Philosophy*, 5 vols. (Cambridge: Cambridge University Press, 1922–1955) 5:20.

48. Dasgupta, *History of Indian Philosophy*, 1:71.

49. Mircea Eliade, *Yoga, Immortality and Freedom*, trans. Willard R. Trask (Princeton: Princeton University Press, Bollingen Series Vol. 76, 1958) 200.

50. Banerji, *Brief History of Tantra Literature*, 8.

51. Sudhir Kakar, "Tantra and Tāntric Healing" in *Shamans, Mystics and Doctors: A Psychological Inquiry into India and its Healing Traditions* (Chicago: University of Chicago Press, 1982, 1991) 151.

52. Banerji, *Brief History of Tantra Literature*, 25.

53. Kakar, *Shamans, Mystics and Doctors*, 154.

54. Manoranjan Basu, *Fundamentals of the Philosophy of Tantras* (Calcutta: Mira Basu Publishers, 1986) 136.

55. Lalan Prasad Singh, *Tantra, Its Mystic and Scientific Basis* (Delhi: Concept Publishing, 1976) 116 n12.

56. Banerji, *Brief History of Tantra Literature*, 122–23.

57. Singh, *Tantra, its Mystic and Scientific Basis*, 128.

58. Eliot Deutsch, *Advaita Vedānta, A Philosophical Reconstruction* (Honolulu: University of Hawaii Press, 1969, 1980) 30.

59. Deutsch, *Advaita Vedanta*, 32.

60. Kamalakar Mishra, *Significance of the Tāntric Tradition* (Varanasi: Arddhanarisvara Publications, 1981) 44.

61. Eliade, *Yoga, Immortality and Freedom*, 206.

62. Mishra, *Significance of the Tāntric Tradition*, 22–24, 32.

63. Singh, *Tantra, Its Mystic and Scientific Basis*, 43.

64. Singh, *Tantra, Its Mystic and Scientific Basis*, 140.

65. *Ratnasāra Tantra*, cited in Pragna R. Shah, *Tantra, Its Therapeutic Aspect* (Calcutta: Punthi Pustak, 1987) 12.

66. Eliade, *Yoga, Immortality and Freedom*, 227.

67. Eliade, *Yoga, Immortality and Freedom*, 228.

68. Eliade, *Yoga, Immortality and Freedom*, 235–36, 239–40.

69. Mishra, *Significance of the Tāntric Tradition*, 63–64.

70. Shah, *Tantra, its Therapeutic Aspect*, 79.

71. *Oxford English Dictionary* [*OED*], 2nd edition, 20 vols. Prepared by J. A. Simpson and E. S. C. Weiner (Oxford: Clarendon Press, 1989) s. v. 'sublimate.'

72. Singh, *Tantra, Its Mystic and Scientific Basis*, 140.

73. Mishra, *Significance of the Tāntric Tradition*, 77.

74. Kakar, *Shamans, Mystics and Doctors*, 224.

75. R. K. Sharma and Bhagwan Dash, *Caraka-saṃhitā of Agniveśa, Text with English Translation and Critical Exposition Based on Cakrapāṇidatta's Āyurveda Dīpikā*, 3 volumes (Varanasi: Chowkhambha Sanskrit Series Office, 1976, 1977, 1988) xxii.

76. Vasant Lad, *Āyurveda, The Science of Self-Healing* (Santa Fe, NM: Lotus Press, 1984, 113–14.

77. Gerald James Larson, "Āyurveda and the Classical Hindu Philosophical Systems," in *Body as Self*, ed. Kasulis et al., 106. First published in *Philosophy East and West* 37 (3) July 1987.

78. Jean Filliozat, *The Classical Doctrine of Indian Medicine* (Delhi: Munshiram Manoharlal, 1964) 26.

79. Cromwell Crawford, "Āyurveda: The Science of Long Life in Contemporary Perspective," in *Eastern and Western Approaches to Healing*, ed. Anees A. Sheikh and Katharina S. Sheikh (New York: John Wiley and Sons, 1989) 11–12.

80. Zimmermann, *The Jungle and the Aroma of Meats*, x.

81. Plato, *Timaeus*, 89c. *Collected Dialogues of Plato*.

82. *Huang Ti Nei Ching Su Wên: The Yellow Emperor's Classic of Internal Medicine*, trans. Ilza Veith (Berkeley: University of California Press, 1972) 97.

83. Larson, "Āyurveda and the Hindu Philosophical Systems," in *Self as Body*, ed. Kasulis et al., 108.

84. Vaidya Bhagwan Dash and Acarya Manfred Junius, *A Handbook of Āyurveda* (New Delhi: Concept Publishing Co., 1983) 11.

85. Crawford, "Āyurveda: The Science of Long Life," in *Eastern and Western Approaches to Healing*, ed. Sheikh and Sheikh, 15.

86. Crawford, "Āyurveda: The Science of Long Life," 15.

87. Zimmermann, *The Jungle and the Aroma of Meats*, 159, 205.

88. Zimmermann, *The Jungle and the Aroma of Meats*, 168.

CHAPTER 2: MEANINGS OF HEALTH IN ĀYURVEDA

1. David M. Eisenberg, MD, and Ronald C. Kessler, Cindy Foster, Frances E. Norlock, David R. Calkins, and Thomas L. Delbanco. "Unconventional Medicine in the United States: Prevalence, Costs, and Patterns of Use," *New England Journal of Medicine* 328 (Jan. 28, 1993) 246–52. See also Oscar Janiger, MD, and Philip Goldberg, "Daring to Be Different," *Hippocrates* 7 (6 June 1993) 42–48.

2. Gerald James Larson, "Āyurveda and the Hindu Philosophical Systems," in *Self as Body in Asian Theory and Practice*, ed. Thomas P. Kasulis, Roger T. Ames, and Wimal Dissanayake (Albany: State University of New York Press, 1993) 104. First published in *Philosophy East and West* 37 (3) July 1987.

3. Quotations from the *Caraka-saṃhitā* and *Ayurveda-dīpikā* are from the English translation of the *Caraka-saṃhitā* by R. K. Sharma and Bhagwan Dash, 3 vols. (Varanasi: Chowkhamba Sanskrit Series, Vol. 94, 1976, 1977, 1988), in consultation with the translation of P. V. Sharma: *Caraka-saṃhitā: Agniveśa's treatise refined and annotated by Charaka and redacted by Dṛḍhabala*, 4 vols. (Varanasi: Chaukhamba Orientalia, Jaikrishnadas Āyurveda Series Vol. 36, 1994, 1995).

4. "Constitution of the World Health Organization," in *Concepts of Health and Disease, Interdisciplinary Perspectives*, ed. Arthur L. Caplan, H. Tristam Engelhardt, Jr., and James J. McCartney (Reading, MA: Addison-Wesley Publishing Co., 1981) 83.

5. Susan Sontag, *Illness as Metaphor* (New York: Random House, Vintage Books, 1977, 1979) 3.

6. Deepak Chopra, *Perfect Health* (New York: Harmony Books, 1991) 3.

7. Deepak Chopra, *Quantum Healing: Exploring the Frontiers of Mind/Body Medicine* (New York: Bantam Books, 1989) 110.

8. Chopra, *Quantum Healing*, 131.

9. Caroline Whitbeck, "A Theory of Health" in *Concepts of Health and Disease*, ed. Caplan et al., 613.

10. Paul Tillich, "The Meaning of Health," in *Religion and Medicine: Essays on Meaning, Values and Health*, ed. David Belgum (Ames: The Iowa State University Press, 1967) 5.

11. Friedrich Nietzsche, *The Gay Science* [1882], trans. Walter Kaufmann (New York: Random House, 1974) 177.

12. H. Tristam Engelhardt, Jr., "The Concepts of Health and Disease," in *Concepts of Health and Disease*, ed. Caplan et al., 42–43.

13. "Constitution of the World Health Organization" in *Concepts of Health and Disease*, ed. Caplan et al., 83.

14. Christopher Boorse, "Health as a Theoretical Concept," *Philosophy of Science* 44 (1977) 542.

15. Georg Canguilhem, *On the Normal and the Pathological*, trans. Carolyn R. Fawcett (New York: Zone Books, 1989) 200–201.

16. Rudolph Virchow, "Natural Scientific Methods and Standpoints in Therapy," trans. S. G. M. Engelhardt. In *Concepts of Health and Disease*, ed. Caplan et al., 188.

17. Drew Leder, *The Absent Body* (Chicago and London: University of Chicago Press, 1990) 89.

18. Burton Watson, trans. *The Complete Works of Chuang Tzu* (New York: Columbia University Press, 1968) 361.

19. Yoel Hoffmann, *Japanese Death Poems, Written by Zen Monks and Haiku Poets on the Verge of Death* (Rutland, VT, and Tokyo: Charles E. Tuttle, 1986).

20. Vaidya Bhagwan Dash and Acarya Manfred M. Junius, *A Handbook of Ayurveda* (New Delhi: Concept Publishing Co., 1983) 2.

21. Vasant Lad, "The Concept of Disease Process," Lecture 4, *Lectures in Āyurveda*, audio cassette series, 6 volumes (Albuquerque, NM: The Ayurvedic Institute, no date).

22. Dash and Junius, *A Handbook of Āyurveda,* 2.

23. René Dubos, "Hippocrates in Modern Dress" in *Ways of Health: Holistic Approaches to Ancient and Contemporary Medicine*, ed. David S. Sobel (New York and London: Harcourt Brace Jovanovich, 1979) 208.

24. Howard Brody and David S. Sobel, "A Systems View of Health and Disease," in *Ways of Health: Holistic Approaches to Ancient and Contemporary Medicine*, ed. David S. Sobel (New York and London: Harcourt Brace Jovanovich, 1979) 93n.

25. Brody and Sobel, "A Systems View of Health and Disease," in *Ways of Health,* ed. Sobel, 91.

26. Brody and Sobel, "A Systems View of Health and Disease," in *Ways of Health,* ed. Sobel, 93.

27. Jozsef Kovács, "Concepts of Health and Disease," *Journal of Medicine and Philosophy* 14 (1989) 261.

28. Kovács, "Concepts of Health and Disease," 262.

29. Richard B. Carter, *Descartes' Medical Philosophy: The Organic Solution to the Mind-Body Problem* (Baltimore, MD, and London: The Johns Hopkins University Press, 1983) 1–4.

30. Abraham Maslow and Bela Mittelmann, "The Meaning of 'Healthy' (Normal) and of 'Sick' (Abnormal)" in *Concepts of Health and Disease*, ed. Caplan et al., 47.

31. John Sanford, *Healing and Wholeness* (New York: Paulist Press, 1967) 13.

32. Boorse, "Health as a Theoretical Concept," 545.

33. Zimmermann, *The Jungle and the Aroma of Meats: An Ecological Theme in Hindu Medicine* (Berkeley: University of California Press, 1987) 24.

34. Zimmermann, *The Jungle and the Aroma of Meats*, 24.

35. Zimmermann, *The Jungle and the Aroma of Meats*, 24–25.

36. Zimmermann, *The Jungle and the Aroma of Meats*, 9.

37. Vaidya Bhagwan Dash and Vaidya Lalitesh Kashyap, *Basic Principles of Ayurveda* (New Delhi: Concept Publishing Co., 1980) 234; cited in Dash and Junius, *A Handbook of Ayurveda*, 34.

38. Boorse, "Health as a Theoretical Concept," 542–73.

39. Mervyn Susser, "Ethical Components in the Definition of Health," in *Concepts of Health and Disease*, ed. Caplan et al., 95.

40. Birgit Heyn, *Ayurveda, The Indian Art of Natural Medicine and Life Extension* (Rochester, VT: Healing Arts Press, 1990) 43.

41. Heyn, *Ayurveda, The Indian Art of Natural Medicine*, 47.

42. Francis Zimmermann, *The Jungle and the Aroma of Meats*, 169.

43. Zimmermann, *The Jungle and the Aroma of Meats*, 120.

44. Daniel C. Tabor, "Ripe and Unripe: Concepts of Health and Sickness in Ayurvedic Medicine," *Social Science and Medicine* 15B (1981) 442.

45. Tabor, "Ripe and Unripe," 446.

46. Tabor, "Ripe and Unripe," 447; Lad, *Ayurveda, the Science of Self-Healing*, 79.

47. Friedrich Nietzsche, *The Will to Power* [1901], trans. Walter Kaufmann and R. J. Hollingdale (New York: Vintage Books, 1967) 29.

48. Nietzsche, *The Gay Science*, 177.

49. Leder, *The Absent Body*,160.

50. Leder, *The Absent Body*, 79.

51. Leon R. Kass, "Regarding the End of Medicine and the Pursuit of Health," in *Concepts of Health and Disease*, ed. Caplan et al., 17.

52. Zimmermann, *The Jungle and the Aroma of Meats*, 25.

53. *American Heritage Dictionary*, Appendix: "Indo-European Roots" (Boston: Houghton Mifflin, 1981) 1520, s. v. 'kailo-.'

54. Sobel, *Ways of Health*, 17.

55. Kass, "Regarding the End of Medicine and the Pursuit of Health," in *Concepts of Health and Disease*, ed. Caplan et al., 17.

56. C. G. Jung, *Modern Man in Search of a Soul*, trans. W. S. Dell and Cary F. Baynes (New York and London: Harcourt Brace Jovanovich, 1933) 202.

57. Sanford, *Healing and Wholeness*, 16.

58. *American Heritage Dictionary*, Appendix: "Indo-European Roots," 1545, s. v. 'tag-.'

59. Leder, *The Absent Body*, 83.

60. Leder, *The Absent Body*, 71.

61. Leder, *The Absent Body*, 84, 86–87.

62. G. W. F. Hegel, *Philosophy of Nature*, trans. Michael John Perry (New York: Humanities Press, 1970) Vol. 3:193; cited in Leder, *The Absent Body*, 88.

63. Leder, *The Absent Body*, 91.

64. Eliot Deutsch, *Creative Being, The Crafting of Person and World* (Honolulu: University of Hawaii Press, 1992) 33.

65. Deutsch, *Creative Being*, 235–36 n1. See Herbert Fingarette, *Self-Deception* (New York: Humanities Press, 1969).

66. Deutsch, *Creative Being*, 236 n2.

67. Rudolf Virchow, cited in Carter, *Descartes' Medical Philosophy*, 5–6.

68. Wang Yang-ming, *Instructions for Practical Living and other Neo-*

Confucian Writings, trans. and ed. Wing-tsit Chan (New York: Columbia University Press, 1963) 273; cited in Leder, *The Absent Body*, 164.

69. Leder, *The Absent Body*, 161–73.

70. René Descartes, *The Philosophical Writings of Descartes*, 2 volumes, trans. John Cottingham, Robert Stoothoff, and Dugald Murdoch, 2 vols. (London and New York: Cambridge University Press, 1984, 1985): *Meditations on First Philosophy*, 2:33.

71. Carter, *Descartes' Medical Philosophy*, 235.

72. Carter, *Descartes' Medical Philosophy*, 236.

73. Gerald James Larson, "Life Science (*Āyurveda*) Old and New: In Search of New Agendas for Healing." Paper presented at University of Hawaii Center for South Asian Studies 10th Spring Symposium: *Health and Healing in Medical Systems of South Asia* (Honolulu, April 12, 1993).

74. Zimmermann, *The Jungle and the Aroma of Meats*, 20.

75. Chopra, *Perfect Health*, 309–310.

76. Claude Bernard, cited in Chopra, *Creating Health* (Boston: Houghton Mifflin, 1987, 1990) 181.

77. Chopra, *Creating Health*, 83.

78. Deepak Chopra, *Ageless Body, Timeless Mind* (New York: Harmony Books, 1993) 318.

79. Walter Kaufmann, *Nietzsche: Philosopher, Psychologist, Antichrist* (Princeton, NJ: Princeton University Press, 1968) 130.

80. Deutsch, *Creative Being*, 155.

81. Deutsch, *Creative Being*, 32.

82. Plato, *Symposium*, 208e-209b. In *Collected Dialogues of Plato*, ed. Edith Hamilton and Huntington Cairns (Princeton, NJ: Princeton University Press, 1961).

83. Erik H. Erikson, *Childhood and Society* (New York: W. W Norton, 1950, 1963) 266–67.

84. Maslow and Mittelmann, "The Meaning of 'Healthy,'" in *Concepts of Health*, ed. Caplan et al., 49.

85. Tillich, "The Meaning of Health," 4.

86. Nietzsche, *The Gay Science*, 177.

87. Ingmar Pörn, "An Equilibrium Model of Health," in *Health, Disease, and Causal Explanation in Medicine*, ed. L. Nordenfelt and B. I. B. Lindahl (Dordrecht and Boston: D. Reidel Publishing Co., 1984) 5.

88. Wilhelm Halbfass, *Tradition and Reflection, Explorations in Indian Thought* (Albany: State University of New York Press, 1991) 249.

89. Sureśvara's *Sambandhavārtikka* (the introduction to his commentary on Śaṅkara's *Bṛhadāraṇyakopaniṣad-bhāṣya*) verse 28; cited in Halbfass, *Tradition and Reflection*, 251.

90. Deutsch, *Creative Being*, 40, 34.

91. Engelhardt, "The Concepts of Health and Disease" in *Concepts of Health and Disease*, ed. Caplan et al., 42.

92. Cromwell Crawford, "Āyurveda: The Science of Long Life in Contemporary Perspective," in *Eastern and Western Approaches to Healing*, ed. Anees A. Sheikh and Katherina S. Sheikh (New York: John Wiley and Sons, 1989) 30.

93. Kenneth Zysk, *Asceticism and Healing in Ancient India: Medicine and the Buddhist Monastery* (New York and Oxford: Oxford University Press, 1991) 6–7. See also Debiprasad Chattopadhyaya, *Science and Society in Ancient India* (Calcutta: Research India Publications, 1977).

94. See, for example, *Caraka-saṃhitā* Vol. 1 *(Sūtra-sthāna)*, chapters 5–7.

95. Chopra, *Perfect Health*, 201.

96. Chopra, *Perfect Health*, 199–211.

97. David L. Wheeler, "A Physician-Anthropologist Examines What Ails America's Medical System," *Chronicle of Higher Education* 39 (39), June 2, 1993, A6–7. Konner's book is *Medicine at the Crossroads: The Crisis in healthcare* (Pantheon).

98. Friedrich Nietzsche, *The Will to Power*, 520.

99. Friedrich Nietzsche, *The Gay Science*, 346.

CHAPTER 3: CLASSICAL YOGA AS A RELIGIOUS THERAPEUTIC

1. *American Heritage Dictionary,* Appendix: "Indo-European Roots" (Boston: Houghton Mifflin, 1981) 1550, s. v. 'yuj.'

2. Sir Monier Monier-Williams, *A Sanskrit-English Dictionary* (London: Oxford University Press, 1899, 1974) 856, s. v. 'yoga.'

3. Surendranath Dasgupta, *A History of Indian Philosophy*, 5 vols. (Cambridge: Cambridge University Press, 1952–1955) 1:226.

4. *Oxford English Dictionary* [*OED*] 2nd edition, 20 vols. Prepared by J. A. Simpson and E. S. C. Weiner (Oxford: Clarendon Press, 1989) 17:568, s. v. 'religion'; *American Heritage Dictionary*, 1526, s. v. 'leig.'

5. Mircea Eliade, *Yoga, Immortality and Freedom*, trans. Willard R. Trask (Princeton, NJ: Princeton University Press [Bollingen Series Vol. 56] 1958, 1973) 5.

6. Eliade, *Yoga, Immortality and Freedom*, 5.

7. Eliade, *Yoga, Immortality and Freedom*, 4

8. Kashi Nath Upadhyaya, *Early Buddhism and the Bhagavadgītā* (Delhi: Motilal Banarsidass, 1971, 1983) 124.

9. Upadhyaya, *Early Buddhism and the Bhagavadgītā*, 122.

10. Upadhyaya, *Early Buddhism and the Bhagavadgītā*, 122–23.

11. Dasgupta, *History of Indian Philosophy*, 2: 443.

12. *Buddhacarita*, 12.17ff; *Saundārmanda* 15–17; *Majjima-nikāya*, 1.164ff, cited in Eliade, *Yoga, Immortality and Freedom*, 162.

13. *Māha-sattipaṭṭhāna-suttanta* (Pondichery: All India Press, 1985) 5.

14. Eliade, *Yoga, Immortality and Freedom*, 210.

15. Georg Feuerstein, *Encyclopedic Dictionary of Yoga* (New York: Paragon, 1990) 150.

16. Main texts of Kuṇḍalinī Yoga are the *Ṣaṭ-cakra-nirūpaṇa* (describing the cakras), the *Pāduka-pañcaka*, "The Fivefold Footstool," and the *Gorakṣa Saṃhitā*.

17. The *Haṭha Yoga Pradīpikā* (fourteenth century C.E.) was written by Svātmārāma Yogīndra, who named as his gūrus the circa 10th-century Tāntric adept Matsyendra, and his disciple Gorakṣa, author of the *Gorakṣa-saṃhitā*.

18. *Haṭha-yoga-saṃhitā* 4.104; *Gheranda-saṃhitā* 1.1; *Śiva-saṃhitā* 5.181.

19. Śri Aurobindo, *The Synthesis of Yoga* (Pondicherry: Śri Aurobindo Ashram, 1971).

20. R. Ravindra, "Is Religion Psychotherapy?" *Religious Studies* 14 (Spring 1978) 396.

21. Ravindra, "Is Religion Psychotherapy?" 14:393.

22. Frank Podgorski, "Sāṃkhya-Yoga Meditation: Psycho-Spiritual Transvaluation," *Journal of Dharma* 2 (April 1977) 158.

23. I. K. Taimni, *The Science of Yoga: The Yoga-Sutras of Patanjali in Sanskrit with transliteration in Roman, translation in English and commentary* (Madras, London, Wheaton, IL: Theosophical Publishing House, 1961) 120.

24. Swami Adidevananda, *Yoga as a Therapeutic Fact* (Mysore: University of Mysore: Prasaranga, 1966) 52.

25. Swami Ramakrishnananda, "Yoga," *Brahmavadin* 1895–1914, vol. 2: *Yoga* (Bangalore: Swami Vivekananda Seva Samithi, 1984) 11.

26. Dasgupta, *History of Indian Philosophy*, 1:266.

27. Halbfass, *Tradition and Reflection, Explorations in Indian Thought* (Albany: State University of New York Press, 1991) 252.

28. B. K. S. Iyengar, *Light on the Yoga Sūtras of Patañjali : Pātañjala Yoga Pradīpikā* (London and San Francisco, CA: Harper Collins 1993) 110–11.

29. Swami Adidevananda, *Yoga as a Therapeutic Fact*, 31.

30. Swami Adidevananda, *Yoga as a Therapeutic Fact*, 15.

31. Dasgupta, *History of Indian Philosophy*, 1:75.

32. S. Cromwell Crawford, *The Evolution of Hindu Ethical Ideals* (Calcutta: Firma K. L. Mukhopadhyay, 1974) 152.

33. Larry Dossey, *Space, Time, and Medicine* (Boulder, CO, and London: Shambhala, 1982) 49–50.

34. Dhirendra Mohan Datta, *The Philosophy of Mahātma Gandhi* (Madison: University of Wisconsin Press, 1953, 1972) 98.

35. Haṭha Yoga's six *kriyās* or cleansing actions involve washing and stimulation (with air, water, or strips of fabric) of various passages of the body (*Haṭha Yoga Pradīpikā*, 2.21–37). For detailed information about the *kriyās* and their variations, see Swami Kuvalayananda and S. L. Vinekar, *Yoga Therapy: Its Basic Principles and Methods* (New Delhi: India Ministry of Health, 1963) 56–74.

36. Śivananda Yoga Vedānta Center, *The Śivananda Companion to Yoga* (New York: Simon and Schuster, 1983) 80.

37. R. S. Khare, "Food with Saints: An Aspect of Hindu Gastrosemantics" in *The Eternal Food, Gastronomic Ideas of Hindus and Buddhists*, ed. R. S. Khare (Albany: State University of New York Press, 1992) 29.

38. R. S. Khare, "Food with Saints," 34.

39. S. Cromwell Crawford, *The Evolution of Hindu Ethical Ideals*, 147.

40. Swami Adidevananda, *Yoga as a Therapeutic Fact*, 37.

41. The *Haṭha Yoga Pradīpikā*, Book One, is a major textual source on *āsana*.

42. B. K. S. Iyengar, *The Tree of Yoga* (Boston: Shambhala, 1989) 55.

43. Iyengar, *Tree of Yoga*, 54–55.

44. Iyengar, *Tree of Yoga*, 56.

45. Iyengar, *Tree of Yoga*, 8, 50–60.

46. Swami Vivekananda, *Complete Works*, 8 vols. (Calcutta: Advaita Ashrama, 1847, 1986) 1:137–39.
47. Iyengar, *Light on the Yoga Sūtras*, 150.
48. Eliot Deutsch, *Creative Being: The Crafting of Person and World* (Honolulu: University of Hawaii Press, 1992) 58–69.
49. Vasant Lad, *Āyurveda, The Science of Self-Healing* (Santa Fe, NM: Lotus Press, 1985) 113.
50. Lad, *Āyurveda, The Science of Self-Healing*, 115–25.
51. B. K. S. Iyengar, *Light on Yoga* (New York: Schocken, 1978) 288–306.
52. "*Āsana* or Posture," *Brahmavadin* (1984) 2:250.
53. Book Two of the *Haṭha Yoga Pradīpikā* gives instructions for *prāṇāyāma*, and Book Three describes the *mudrās* or 'seals,' techniques for harnessing and utilizing *prāṇa*. Book Four treats *samādhi*, showing that Haṭha Yoga, like classical Yoga, aims for liberation, though Haṭha is more oriented to body and health.
54. Swami Vivekananda, "Rāja-Yoga" in *Complete Works*, 1:267.
55. Vivekananda, *Complete Works*, 1:147.
56. Vivekananda, *Complete Works*, 1:148.
57. Vivekananda, *Complete Works*, 1:149–51.
58. *OED*, 16:251, s. v. 'spirit.'
59. Vivekananda, *Complete Works*, 1:143–44.
60. Hirendra Nath Sinha, "Prāṇāyāma," *Brahmavadin* (1984) 2:299.
61. Iyengar, *Light on the Yoga Sūtras*, 152.
62. T. V. K. Desikachar, *Religiousness in Yoga, Lectures in Theory and Practice*, ed. Mary Louise Skelton and John Ross Carter (Washington, D. C.: University Press of America, 1980) 163–72.
63. I. K. Taimni, *The Science of Yoga*, 261.
64. Desikachar, *Religiousness in Yoga*, 135–36.
65. See also Baba Hari Dass, *Ashtanga Yoga Primer* (Santa Cruz, CA: Sri Rama Publishing, 1981) 8–9.
66. Desikachar, *Religiousness in Yoga*, 139–43.
67. Sinha,"Prāṇāyāma," *Brahmavadin* (1984) 2:294.
68. Eliade, *Yoga, Immortality and Freedom*, 58.
69. Desikachar, *Religiousness in Yoga*, 152.
70. Sinha, "Pratyāhāra or the Gathering of the Senses," *Brahmavadin* (1984) 2:357.
71. Eliade, *Yoga, Immortality and Freedom*, 98–99, 124.
72. Eliade, *Yoga, Immortality and Freedom*, 70.
73. Iyengar, *Tree of Yoga*, 8, 65.
74. Eliade, *Yoga, Immortality and Freedom*, 77.
75. Iyengar, *Tree of Yoga*, 8–9.
76. Sinha, "Dhyāna or Meditation," *Brahmavadin* 2:373.
77. Sinha, "Dhyāna or Meditation," *Brahmavadin* 2:368.
78. Eliade, *Yoga, Immortality and Freedom*, 72–73.
79. Eliade, *Yoga, Immortality and Freedom*, 78.
80. Iyengar, *Light on the Yoga-Sūtras*, 170.
81. Eliade, *Yoga, Immortality and Freedom*, 80, 82.
82. *OED*, 18:382 s. v. 'trance.'

83. Eliade, *Yoga, Immortality and Freedom*, 78–79.

84. Mircea Eliade, *Shamanism, Archaic Techniques of Ecstasy*, Willard Trask, trans. (Princeton, NJ: Princeton University Press [Bollingen Series Vol. 76], 1964) 5, 107, 417.

85. Sinha, "Samādhi or Hyper-Conscious State of Existence," *Brahmavadin* (1984) 2:392.

86. Dasgupta, *History of Indian Philosophy*, 1: 271.

87. Sinha, "Samādhi," *Brahmavadin* (1984) 2:413.

88. Eliade, *Yoga, Immortality and Freedom*, 91.

89. S. N. Dasgupta, *Yoga Philosophy in Relation to Other Systems of Indian Thought* (Delhi: Motilal Banarsidass, 1930, 1974) 341.

90. Dasgupta, *Yoga as Philosophy and as Religion* (Delhi: Motilal Banarsidass, 1924) 150–53.

91. Dasgupta, *Yoga as Philosophy and Religion*, 117.

92. A. Wezler, "On the Quadruple Division of the Yogaśastra, the Caturvyūhatva of the Cikitāśāstra and the Four Noble Truths of the Buddha," *Indologica Taurensia* 12 (1984) 304.

93. Halbfass, *Tradition and Reflection*, 250.

94. Halbfass, *Tradition and Reflection*, 250.

95. Halbfass, *Tradition and Reflection*, 256.

96. Halbfass, *Tradition and Reflection*, 248.

97. *American Heritage Dictionary*, Appendix: "Indo-European Roots," 1520, s. v. 'kailo-.'

98. *OED*, 14:420, s. v. 'salvation.'

99. *American Heritage Dictionary*, Appendix: "Indo-European Roots," 1537, s. v. 'sak-.'

100. *OED*, 14:338–39, s. v. 'sacred.'

101. Mary Douglas, *Purity and Danger: An Analysis of Concepts of Pollution and Taboo* (New York: Frederick A. Praeger, 1966) 35.

102. V. S. Apte, *English-Sanskrit Dictionary* (New Delhi: Publications India, reprint 1989) 199, s. v. 'free.'

CHAPTER 4: TANTRA AND AESTHETIC THERAPEUTICS

1. Mircea Eliade, *Yoga, Immortality and Freedom*, trans. Willard R. Trask (Princeton, NJ: Princeton University Press [Bollingen Series Vol. 56], 1958, 1973) 230.

2. Sir John Woodroffe, *Shakti and Shakta* (Madras and London, 1929) 7; cited in Heinrich Zimmer, *Philosophies of India*, ed. Joseph Campbell (New York: Pantheon Press [Bollingen Series Vol. 26, 1951) 570.

3. Manoranjan Basu, *Fundamentals of the Philosophy of Tantras* (Calcutta: Mira Basu Publishers, 1986), 72.

4. S. C. Banerji, *Brief History of Tantra Literature* (Calcutta: Naya Prokash, 1988) 32; Basu, *Fundamentals of the Philosophy of Tantras*, 622.

5. M. P. Pandit, *Lights on the Tantra* (Madras: Ganesh and Co., 1977) 9.

6. Sudhir Kakar, *Shamans, Mystics and Doctors: An Inquiry into India and Its Healing Traditions* (Chicago, IL: University of Chicago Press, 1982, 1991) 166–68.

7. Kamalakar Mishra, *Significance of the Tāntric Tradition* (Varanasi: Arddhanarīśvara Publications, 1981) 3–7.

8. Sir John Woodroffe (Arthur Avalon), *Introduction to Tantra Shastra* (Madras: Ganesh and Co., 1913, 1952) 21.

9. Eliade, *Yoga, Immortality and Freedom*, 244–45.

10. Eliade, *Yoga, Immortality and Freedom*, 209–11.

11. Pragna R. Shah, *Tantra, its Therapeutic Aspect* (Calcutta: Punthi Pustak, 1987), 40.

12. Louis Renou, *L'Inde Classique*, 568, cited in Eliade, *Yoga, Immortality and Freedom*, 219.

13. See, for example, *Śrī-Cakra, its Yantra, Mantra, and Tantra*, by S. K. Ramachandra Rao (Bangalore: Kalpatharu Research Academy, 1982).

14. Eliade, *Yoga, Immortality and Freedom*, 225–26.

15. John Thomas Casey, Drawing of *Śrā Yantra*, and interview by author. Honolulu, HI, March 1994.

16. Kakar, *Shamans, Mystics and Doctors*, 154.

17. Mishra, *Significance of the Tāntric Tradition*, 62.

18. Shah, *Tantra, its Therapeutic Aspect*, 15.

19. Sir John Woodroffe, *Introduction to Tantra Shastra*, 112–13.

20. Eliade, *Yoga, Immortality and Freedom*, 259.

21. Eliade, *Yoga, Immortality and Freedom*, 270–71.

22. *Kulārṇava Tantra* 10:6, cited in Mishra, *Significance of the Tāntric Tradition*, 65–66.

23. Eliade, *Yoga, Immortality and Freedom*, 267–68.

24. Banerji, *Brief History of Tantra Literature*, 18.

25. *Kulārṇava Tantra* 10:5; cited in Mishra, *Significance of the Tāntric Tradition*, 65–66, 69.

26. Mishra, *Significance of the Tāntric Tradition*, 68–71.

27. *Tantratattva (Principles of Tantra): The Tantratattva of Śrīyukta Śiva Chandra Vidyarāṇava Bhattacārya Mahodaya*, 2 vols., ed. Arthur Avalon (Sir John Woodroffe). (Madras: Ganesh and Co., 1914, 1960) 544; Zimmer, *Philosophies of India*, 572–73.

28. Kakar, *Shamans, Mystics and Doctors*, 153.

29. Pandit, *Lights on the Tantras*, 6.

30. *The Yoga-Upaniṣads*, trans. T. R. Srīnivasa Ayyaṅgar (Madras: Adyar Library, Vasanta Press, 1938).

31. Surendranath Dasgupta, *A History of Indian Philosophy*, 5 vols. (Cambridge: Cambridge University Press, 1922–55) 1:228–29.

32. Lalan Prasad Singh, *Tantra, Its Mystic and Scientific Basis* (Delhi: Concept Publishing Co., 1976) 137.

33. Mishra, *Significance of the Tāntric Tradition*, 47–48.

34. Shah, *Tantra, its Therapeutic Aspect*, 3, 30.

35. Basu, *Fundamentals of the Philosophy of Tantras*, 80.

36. Arthur Avalon (Sir John Woodroffe) *The Serpent Power* (*Ṣaṭ-cakra-nirūāpaṇa* and *Pādukā-pañcaka*) (Madras: Ganesh and Co., 1918, 1964) 222.

37. Shah, *Tantra, its Therapeutic Aspect*, 80.

38. *Tantraloka* 2; cited in Singh, *Tantra, Its Mystic and Scientific Basis*, 65.

39. See also Harish Johari, *Chakras, Energy Centers of Transformation* (Rochester, VT: Destiny Books, 1987).

40. Woodroffe, *The Serpent Power*, 228.

41. Sir John Woodroffe (Arthur Avalon), *The Garland of Letters* (*Varṇamālā*), *Studies in the Mantra śāstra* (Madras: Ganesh and Co.,1922, 1994) 232.

42. Eliade, *Yoga, Immortality and Freedom*, 212.

43. Kakar, *Shamans, Mystics and Doctors*, 172.

44. Woodroffe, *The Garland of Letters* (*Varṇamālā*), 218–19, 232; Woodroffe, *Introduction to Tantra Shastra*, 81–82.

45. Eliade, *Yoga, Immortality and Freedom*, 215.

46. Eliade, *Yoga, Immortality and Freedom*, 212–13.

47. The Sanskrit alphabet consists of the forty-nine primordial *bījas* or seed-sounds, arranged in a logical matrix. The matrix of the Sanskrit alphabet presents a set of pure and basic sounds, systematically arranged according to factors such as the point in the mouth where the sound is articulated (e.g., the guttural *ka* is articulated in the throat, and the labial *ma*, at the lips).

48. Banerji, *Brief History of Tantra Literature*, 116.

49. Woodroffe, *Introduction to Tantra Shastra*, 107.

50. Singh, *Tantra, its Mystic and Scientific Basis*, 79.

51. Woodroffe, *The Garland of Letters* (*Varṇamālā*), 233.

52. Basu, *Fundamentals of the Philosophy of Tantras*, 622–23.

53. Eliade, *Yoga, Immortality and Freedom*, 215.

54. Eliade, *Yoga, Immortality and Freedom*, 215.

55. Singh, *Tantra, its Mystic and Scientific Basis*, 96.

56. *Vakyapadīya* 1:5,14; cited by Harold Coward, "The Meaning and Power of Mantras in Bhartṛhari's *Vakyapadīya*," in *Understanding Mantras*, ed. Harvey P. Alper (Albany: State University of New York Press, 1989) 172–73.

57. Shah, *Tantra, Its Therapeutic Value*, 114–15.

58. Kakar, *Shamans, Mystics and Doctors*, 172–73. *Om* as a mantra's opening sound signifies the aim of peaceful state, while *Krau* signifies the goal of a psychic state of active struggle.

59. Kakar, *Shamans, Mystics, and Doctors*, 174.

60. Harold Coward, "The Meaning and Power of Mantras in Bhartṛhari's *Vakyapadīya*" in *Understanding Mantras*, ed. Alper, 173–74.

61. *Oxford English Dictionary* [*OED*] 2nd edition, 20 vols., prepared by J. A. Simpson and E. S. C. Weiner. (Oxford: Clarendon Press, 1989) s. v. 'aesthetic.'

62. Avalon (Woodroffe) *Great Liberation* (Madras: Ganesh and Co., 1913, 1953) 65 n4.

63. Basu, *Fundamentals of the Philosophy of Tantras*, 82.

64. Eliade, *Yoga, Immortality and Freedom*, 206.

65. Kakar, *Shamans, Mystics and Doctors*, 166.

66. Shah, *Tantra, its Therapeutic Aspect*, 3.

67. Shah, *Tantra, its Therapeutic Aspect*, 51–54.

68. Vyaas Houston, "Sanskrit, Planetary Language?" in *Devavānī: Sanskrit, Sacred Language, and Self Knowledge* (Warwick, NY: American Sanskrit Institute, 1993) 10.

69. Shah, *Tantra, its Therapeutic Aspect*, 54.

70. *Nāda-bindupaniṣad* 43. *The Yoga-Upaniṣads*, trans. T. R. Śrīnivasa Ayyaṅgar, 178.

71. *Yoga-śikhopaniṣad*, 3:1–5. *Yoga-Upaniṣads*, trans. Ayyaṅgar, 366–68.

72. Lewis Rowell, *Music and Musical Thought in Early India* (Chicago and London: University of Chicago Press, 1992) 10, 166–67.

73. *The Stanzas on Vibration: The Spaṇḍakārikā with Four Commentaries*, trans. Mark S. G. Dyczkowski (Albany: State University of New York Press, 1992)105.

74. Harold G. Coward, "The Spiritual Power of Oral and Written Scripture," in *Silence, the Word and the Sacred*, ed. E. D. Blodgett and H. G. Coward (Waterloo, Ontario, Canada: Wilfred Laurier Press, 1989) 113.

75. Harold G. Koenig, *Is Religion Good for Your Health? The Effects of Religion on Mental and Physical Health* (Binghamton, NY: The Haworth Pastoral Press, 1997) 81–82.

76. James K. McNeley, *Holy Wind in Navajo Philosophy* (Tucson: University of Arizona Press, 1981) 1.

77. Gary Witherspoon, *Language and Art in the Navajo Universe* (Ann Arbor: University of Michigan Press, 1977) 61; cited in McNeley, *Holy Wind in Navajo Philosophy*, 58.

78. Johnny Moses (*Whisstemenee:* Walking Medicine Robe), "Northwest Coast Medicine Teachings: An Interview with Johnny Moses" by Timothy White. *Shaman's Drum* (Spring 1991) 36–43.

79. Johnny Moses, "Native Northwest Coast Song and Drum." Lecture/presentation, Southern Illinois University, Edwardsville, June 14, 1996.

80. Johnny Moses, SiSíWiss Medicine Teachings. First Unitarian Church of Honolulu, Honolulu, Hawaii, May 1993.

81. Swami Prajñānānanda, *A Historical Study of Indian Music* (1975) xxviii, cited in Shah, *Tantra: Its Therapeutic Aspect*, 60–61.

82. William K. Powers, *Sacred Language, The Nature of Supernatural Discourse in Lakota* (Norman: University of Oklahoma Press, 1986) 6, 46–47.

83. Powers, *Sacred Language*, 66–67.

84. Riley Lee, Lecture/performance on the *shakuhachi* flute, East-West Center, Honolulu, Hawaii, October 1993.

85. Vyaas Houston, "The Yoga of Learning Sanskrit," in *Devavānī*, 18.

86. Houston, "Sanskrit—Planetary Language?" in *Devavānī*, 10.

87. Vyaas Houston, "Sanskrit as Spiritual Practice," *Yoga International* (May/June 1992) 30–35. In *Devavānī*, 50.

88. Coward, "Spiritual Power of Oral and Written Scripture," 126.

89. Coward, "Spiritual Power of Oral and Written Scripture," 127.

90. Huston Smith, quoted in *Chant*, National Public Radio Program (Honolulu: University of Hawaii Sinclair Library, audio cassete vol. 975) 1983.

91. Tokeya Inajin (Kevin Locke) and Jim Deerhawk, *Dream Catcher* [audio cassette] (Redway, CA: Earthbeat, 1992) liner notes.

92. Kevin Locke (Tokeya Inajin) in *The Spirit World* [Series: *The American Indians*] (Alexandria, VA: Time-Life Books, 1992) 29.

93. Coward, "Scripture in Hinduism," in *Sacred Word and Sacred Text: Scripture in World Religions*, ed. Harold Coward (Maryknoll, NY: Orbis Books, 1988), 116.

CONCLUSION: *COMMUNITY:* RELATIONALITY IN RELIGIOUS THERAPEUTICS

1. David Frawley and Vasant Lad, *The Yoga of Herbs, An Āyurvedic Guide to Herbal Medicine* (Santa Fe, NM: Lotus Press, 1986) 21–22.

2. David J. Kalupahana, "Buddhism and Healing." Paper presented at The Center for South Asian Studies 10th Spring Symposium: *Healing Systems of South Asia.* (Honolulu: University of Hawaii, April 12, 1993) 12.

3. Kalupahana, "Buddhism and Healing," 13.

4. William R. LaFleur, "Saigyō and the Buddhist Value of Nature" in *Nature in Asian Traditions of Thought: Essays in Environmental Philosophy*, ed. J. Baird Callicott and Roger T. Ames (Albany: State University of New York Press, 1989) 183–209.

5. Kukai, *Kōbō Daishi Zenshū*, ed. Mikkyō Bunka Kenkyūjō (Tokyo, 1964) 2:37; cited in LaFleur, "Saigyō and the Buddhist Value of Nature," 186–87.

6. LaFleur, "Saigyō and the Buddhist Value of Nature," 187.

7. Wallace H. Black Elk, Talks at Church of the Crossroads, Honolulu, Hawaii, March, 1993.

8. Kalupahana, "Buddhism and Healing," 15–16.

9. Kalupahana, "Buddhism and Healing," 14.

10. *Chāndogya Upaniṣad* 1:1.2,5.

11. *Māṇḍūkya Upaniṣad* 1,12.

SOURCES

PRIMARY SOURCES

Atharvaveda

Bloomfield, Maurice, trans. *Hymns of the Atharva-veda*. The Sacred Books of the East, Vol. 42. Edited by F. Max Müller. Delhi: Motilal Banarsidass, 1897, 1964.

Whitney, William Dwight, trans. *Atharva-veda Saṃhitā*, 2 vols. Delhi: Motilal Banarsidass, 1962.

Bhagavadgītā

Radhakrishnan, S. trans. *The Bhagavadgītā*. New York: Harper Colophon Books, 1973.

Sargeant, Winthrop, trans. *The Bhagavadgītā*. Albany: State University of New York Press: 1984.

Caraka-saṃhitā

Sharma, P. V. (Priyavat), ed. and trans. *Caraka-Saṃhitā: Agniveśa's Treatise Refined and Annotated by Caraka and Redacted by Dṛdhabala, Text with English Translation,* 4. vols. Varanasi, Chaukhamba Orientalia [Jaikrishnadas Āyurveda Series Vol. 36], 1994, 1995.

Sharma, Ram Karan and Vaidya Bhagwan Dash, trans. *Carakasaṃhitā* of Agniveśa, *Text with English Translation and Critical Exposition Based on Cakrapāṇidatta's Āyurveda-Dīpikā,* 3 vols. Varanasi: Chowkhamba Sanskrit Series, Vol. 94. 1976, 1977, 1988.

Haṭha Yoga Pradīpikā of Svātmārāma Yogīndra

Sinh, Pancham, trans. *The Haṭha Yoga Pradīpikā*. New Delhi: Munshiram Manoharlal, 1975.

Mahānirvāṇa Tantra

Avalon, Arthur (Sir John Woodroffe), trans. *The Great Liberation*. Madras: Ganesh and Co., 1913, 1953.

Māhasattipaṭṭhāna-suttanta

Pondicherry: All India Press, 1985.

Ṛgveda

Maurer, Walter H. *Pinnacles of India's Past, Selections from the Ṛgveda*. University of Pennsylvania Studies on South Asia, Vol. 2. Amsterdam and Philadelphia, PA: John Benjamins Publishing Co., 1986.

Sāṃkhya-kārikā

Mainkar, T. G., trans. *The Sāṃkhyakārikā of Īśvarakṛṣṇa with the commentary of Gauṣapāda*. Poona: Oriental Book Agency, 1964.

Larson, Gerald James, trans. *Sāṃkhyakārikā of Īśvarakṛṣṇa*. In *Classical Sāṃkhya, An Interpretation of Its History and Meaning*, Appendix B. Delhi: Motilal Banarsidass, 1969, 1979.

Ṣaṭcakra-nirūpaṇa and Pādukā-pañcaka

Avalon, Arthur (Sir John Woodroffe), trans. *The Serpent Power*. Madras: Ganesh and Co., 1918, 1964.

Upaniṣads

Hume, Robert Ernest, trans. *The Thirteen Principle Upanishads*. London, Madras: Oxford University Press, 1921, 1965.

Viveka-cūdāmaṇi of Śaṅkara

Swami Madhavananda, trans. Calcutta: Advaita Ashrama, 1957.

Yoga-sūtras

Fields, Gregory P., *Yoga-sūtras of Patañjali,* translation from Sanskrit to English, in *Religious Therapeutics: Body and Health in Yoga and Āyurvedic Medicine,* Ph.D dissertation, University of Hawaii.

Iyengar, B. K. S., trans. *Light on the Yoga Sūtras of Patañjali: Pātañjala Yoga Prādipikā*. London, San Francisco: HarperCollins, 1993.

Miller, Barbara Stoler, trans. *Yoga: Discipline of Freedom, The Yoga Sūtra Attributed to Patañjali*. Berkeley: University of California Press, 1995.

Taimni, I. K., trans. *The Science of Yoga: The Yoga-sūtras of Patañjali in Sanskrit with Transliteration in Roman, Translation in English and Commentary.* Madras, London, and Wheaton, Illinois: Theosophical Publishing House, 1961.

Rukmani, T. S. *Yogavārtikka of Vijñānabhiksu: Text with English Translation and Critical Notes along with the Text and English Translation of the Pātañjala Yogasūtras and Vyāsabhāṣya*, 4 vols. New Delhi: Munshiram Manoharlal, 1981, 1983, 1987, 1989.

Yoga-sūtras, Yoga-bhāṣya, and Tattva-vāiśāradī

Prasāda, Rāma, trans. *Patañjali's Yoga-sūtras, with the Commentary of Vyāsa and the Gloss of Vāchaspatimiśra*. New Delhi: Munshiram Manoharlal, 1912, 1978.

Woods, James Haughton. *The Yoga-system of Patañjali: The Yoga-sūtras of Patañjali, the Yoga-bhāshya Attributed to Veda-vyāsa, and the Tattva-vaiśāradī of Vāchaspati-miśra*. Harvard Oriental Series, Vol. 17. Cambridge, Massachusetts: Harvard University Press, 1927.

Yoga Upaniṣads

Ayyaṅgar, T. R. Śrīnivāsa, trans. and Pandit S. Subrammaṇya Śāstrī, ed. *The Yoga-Upaniṣads*. Madras: The Adyar Library, Vasanta Press, 1938.

SECONDARY SOURCES

Reference Works

American Heritage Dictionary, Appendix: "Indo-European Roots." Boston: Houghton Mifflin, 1981.

Apte, V. S. *English-Sanskrit Dictionary*. New Delhi: Publications India, reprint 1989.

MacDonnell, Arthur Anthony. *A Practical Sanskrit Dictionary*. Oxford and New York: Oxford University Press, 1924, 1990.

Monier-Williams, Monier. *A Sanskrit-English Dictionary*. Oxford: Oxford University Press, 1899, 1974.

Oxford English Dictionary [*OED*] 2nd edition, 20 vols. Prepared by J. A. Simpson and E. S. C. Weiner. Oxford: Clarendon Press, 1989.

Stedman's Medical Dictionary, 25th edition. Edited by William R. Hensyl. Baltimore, Maryland: Williams and Wilkins, 1990.

Whitney, William Dwight. *The Roots, Verb-forms, and Primary Derivatives of the Sanskrit Language*. New Haven, Connecticut: American Oriental Society, 1945.

Books, Articles, Presentations, and Recordings

Adidevananda, Swami. *Yoga as Therapeutic Fact, Special Lectures*. Mysore: University of Mysore, Prasaranga, 1966.

Ames, Roger T. "The Meaning of Body in Classical Chinese Thought." In *Self as Body in Asian Theory and Practice*, ed. Kasulis et al., 157–77. First published in *International Philosophical Quarterly*, 24:1 (March 1984), 39–54.

Aurobindo. *The Synthesis of Yoga*. Pondicherry: Śri Aurobindo Ashram, 1971.

Banerji, S. C. *A Brief History of Tantra Literature*. Calcutta: Naya Prokash, 1988.

Basu, Manoranjan. *Fundamentals of the Philosophy of Tantras*. Calcutta: Mira Basu Publishers, 1986.

Bhattācharya, Śiva Chandra Vidyārṇava. *Principles of Tantra* (*Tantratattva*). Edited by Arthur Avalon (Sir John Woodroffe), 2 vols. Madras: Ganesh and Co., 1914, 1960.

Bible: *Holy Bible*, King James Version. Grand Rapids, Michigan: Zondervan Bible Publishers, 1989.

Black Elk, Wallace H. Lectures at Church of the Crossroads. Honolulu, Hawaii, March 1993.

Boorse, Christopher, "Health as a Theoretical Concept." *Philosophy of Science* 44 (1977): 542–573.

Brahmavadin 1895–1914, Vol. 2: *Yoga*. Bangalore: Swami Vivekananda Seva Samithi, 1984.

Brody, Howard and David S. Sobel, "A Systems View of Health and Disease." In *Ways of Health*, ed. Sobel, 87–104.

Canguilhem, Georg. *On the Normal and the Pathological*, trans. Carolyn R. Fawcett. New York: Zone Books, 1989. First published as *Le normal et la Pathologique* by Presses Universitaires de France, 1966.

Caplan, Arthur L., H. Tristam Engelhardt, and James J. McCartney, eds. *Concepts of Health and Disease: Interdisciplinary Perspectives.* Reading, Massachusetts: Addison-Wesley Publishing Co., 1981.

Carter, Richard B. *Descartes' Medical Philosophy: The Organic Solution to the Mind-Body Problem.* Baltimore, Maryland, and London: The Johns Hopkins University Press, 1983.

Casey, John Thomas. Drawing of *Śrī Yantra*, and interview by author. Honolulu, Hawaii: March 1994.

Chattopadhyaya, Debiprasad. *Science and Society in Ancient India.* Calcutta: Research India Publications, 1977.

Chopra, Deepak. *Ageless Body, Timeless Mind.* New York: Harmony Books, 1993.

———. *Creating Health. How to Wake Up the Body's Intelligence.* Boston: Houghton Mifflin, 1987, 1990.

———. *Perfect Health: The Complete Mind/Body Guide.* New York: Harmony Books, 1991.

———. *Quantum Healing: Exploring the Frontiers of Mind/Body Medicine.* New York: Bantam Books, 1989.

Coward, Harold. "The Meaning and Power of Mantras in Bhartṛhari's *Vākyapadīya.*" In *Understanding Mantras*, edited by Harvey P. Alper. Albany: State University of New York Press, 1989.

———. "Scripture in Hinduism." In *Sacred Word and Sacred Text, Scripture in World Religions*, edited by Harold Coward, 105–29. Maryknoll, New York: Orbis Books, 1988.

———. "The Spiritual Power of Oral and Written Scripture." In *Silence, the Word and the Sacred*, edited by E. D. Blodgett and H. G. Coward, 111–37. Waterloo, Ontario, Canada: Wilfred Laurier University Press for the Calgary Institute for the Humanities, 1989.

Crawford, S. Cromwell. "Āyurveda: The Science of Long Life in Contemporary Perspective." In *Eastern and Western Approaches to Healing*, ed. Sheikh and Sheikh, 3–32.

———. *The Evolution of Hindu Ethical Ideals.* Calcutta: Firma K. L. Mukhopadhyay, 1974.

Dasgupta, Surendranath. *A History of Indian Philosophy*, 5 vols. Cambridge: Cambridge University Press, 1922–55.

———. *The Study of Patañjali.* Calcutta: University of Calcutta Press, 1920.

———. *Yoga as Philosophy and as Religion.* Delhi: Motilal Banarsidass, 1924.

———. *Yoga Philosophy in Relation to other Systems of Indian Thought.* Delhi: Motilal Banarsidass, 1930, 1974.

Dash, Vaidya Bhagwan, and Acarya Manfred M. Junius, *A Handbook of Ayurveda.* New Delhi: Concept Publishing Co., 1983.

Dass, Baba Hari. *Ashtanga Yoga Primer.* Santa Cruz, California: Sri Rama Publishing, 1981.

Datta, Dhirendra Mohan. *The Philosophy of Mahatma Gandhi.* Madison: University of Wisconsin Press, 1953, 1972.

Descartes, René. *The Philosophical Writings of Descartes*, 2 vols. Translated by John Cottingham, Robert Stoothoff, and Dugald Murdoch. Cambridge: Cambridge University Press, 1985.

Desikachar, T. K. V. *Religiousness in Yoga: Lectures on Theory and Practice*. Edited by Mary Louise Skelston and John Ross Carter. Washington D. C.: University Press of America, 1969.

Deutsch, Eliot, *Advaita Vedānta, A Philosophical Reconstruction*. Honolulu: An East-West Center Book, University of Hawaii Press, 1969, 1980.

———. *Creative Being, The Crafting of Person and World*. Honolulu: University of Hawaii Press, 1992.

Dissanayake, Wimal. Introduction to Part Two: "The Body in Indian Theory and Practice." In *Self as Body*, ed. Kasulis et al., 39–44.

Dossey, Larry. *Space, Time and Medicine*. Boulder, Colorado, and London: Shambhala, 1982.

Douglas, Mary. *Purity and Danger: An Analysis of Concepts of Pollution and Taboo*. New York: Frederick A. Praeger, 1966.

Dubos, René, "Hippocrates in Modern Dress." In *Ways of Health*, ed. Sobel, 205–20.

Dyczkowski, Mark S. G.,trans. *The Stanzas on Vibration: The Spaṇḍakārikā and Four Commentaries*. Albany: State University of New York Press, 1992.

Eisenberg, David M. M. D., Ronald C. Kessler, Cindy Foster, Frances E. Norlock, David R. Calkins, and Thomas L. Delbanco. "Unconventional Medicine in the United States: Prevalence, Costs, and Patterns of Use." *New England Journal of Medicine*, 328 (Jan. 28, 1993) 246–52.

Eliade, Mircea. *Shamanism, Archaic Techniques of Ecstasy*, trans. Willard R. Trask. Princeton, New Jersey: Princeton University Press [Bollingen Series Vol. 76] 1964.

———. *Yoga, Immortality and Freedom*. trans. Willard R. Trask. Princeton, New Jersey: Princeton University Press [Bollingen Series Vol. 56] 1958, 1973.

Engelhardt, H. Tristam, "The Concepts of Health and Disease." In *Concepts of Health and Disease*, ed. Caplan et al., 31–45.

Erickson, Erik H. *Childhood and Society*. New York: W. W. Norton and Co., 1950, 1963.

Feuerstein, Georg. *Encyclopedic Dictionary of Yoga*. New York: Paragon House, 1990.

Filliozat, J. *The Classical Doctrine of Indian Medicine*. New Delhi: Munshiram Manoharlal, 1964.

Frawley, David and Vasant Lad. *The Yoga of Herbs, An Āyurvedic Guide to Herbal Medicine*. Santa Fe, New Mexico: Lotus Press, 1986.

Halbfass, Wilhelm. *Tradition and Reflection: Explorations in Indian Thought*. Albany: State University of New York Press, 1991.

Heyn, Birgit. *Āyurveda, The Indian Art of Natural Medicine and Life Extension*. Rochester, Vermont: Healing Arts Press, 1990. First published as *Die Sanfte Kraft der Indischen Naturheilkunde: Āyurveda* by Scherz Verlag, 1983.

Hoffmann, Yoel. *Japanese Death Poems, Written by Zen Monks and Haiku Poets on the Verge of Death*. Rutland, Vermont, and Tokyo: Charles E. Tuttle Co, 1986.

Houston, Vyaas. *Devavāṇi: Sanskrit, Sacred Language, and Self Knowledge*. Warwick, New York: American Sanskrit Institute, 1993.

———. "Sanskrit as Spiritual Practice." *Yoga International* (May/June 1992) 29–35.

Inajin, Tokeya (Kevin Locke) and Jim Deer Hawk. *Dream Catcher* (audio cassette) Redway, California: Earthbeat, 1992, recording and liner notes.

Iyengar, B. K. S. *Light on Yoga*. London: Unwin, 1976.

———. *Light on the Yoga Sūtras of Patañjali: Pātañjala Yoga Pradīpikā*. London and San Francisco, California: Aquarian Press (HarperCollins), 1993.

———. *The Tree of Yoga*. Boston: Shambhala, 1989.

Janiger, Oscar M. D. and Philip Goldberg. "Daring to be Different." *Hippocrates* 7 (6) June 1993, 42–48. Excerpted from their book, *A Different Kind of Healing*. New York: Putnam, 1993.

Johari, Harish. *Chakras: Energy Centers of Transformation*. Rochester, Vermont: Destiny Books, 1987.

Johnstone, Albert, "The Bodily Nature of The Self or What Descartes Should Have Conceded to Princess Elizabeth." In *Giving the Body Its Due*, ed. Maxine Sheets-Johnstone, 16–47.

Jolly, Julius. *Indian Medicine*, trans. C. G. Kashikar, New Delhi: Concept Publishing Co., 1977.

Jung, C. G. *Modern Man in Search of a Soul*, trans. W. S. Dell and Cary F. Baynes. New York and London: Harcourt Brace Jovanovich, 1933.

Kakar, Sudhir. *Shamans, Mystics and Doctors: An Inquiry into India and its Healing Traditions*. Chicago: University of Chicago Press, 1982, 1991.

Kalupahana, David J. "Buddhism and Healing." Paper presented at the University of Hawaii,Center for South Asian Studies 10th Spring Symposism: *Healing Systems of South Asia*. Honolulu April 12, 1993.

Kass, Leon R. "Regarding the End of Medicine and the Pursuit of Health." In *Concepts of Health and Disease*, ed. Caplan et al., 3–30.

Kasulis, Thomas P., Roger T. Ames, and Wimal Dissanayake, eds. *Self as Body in Asian Theory and Practice*. Albany: State University of New York Press, 1993.

Kaufmann, Walter, *Nietzsche: Philosopher, Psychologist, Antichrist*, 3rd edition. Princeton, New Jersey: Princeton University Press, 1968.

Keswani, N. H. *The Science of Medicine and Physiological Concepts in Ancient and Medieval India*. New Delhi: All-India Institute of Medical Sciences, 1974.

Khare, R. S. "Food with Saints: An Aspect of Hindu Gastrosemantics." In *The Eternal Food, Gastronomic Ideas and Experiences of Hindus and Buddhists*, edited by R. S. Khare, 27–52. Albany: State University of New York Press, 1992.

Koenig, Harold G. *Is Religion Good for Your Health? The Effects of Religion on Mental and Physical Health*. Binghamton, New York: Haworth Pastoral Press, 1997.

Koller, John M. "Human Embodiment: Indian Perspectives." In *Self as Body*, ed. Kasulis et al., 45–58.

Kovács, Jozsef, "Concepts of Health and Disease." *Journal of Medicine and Philosophy* 14 (1989) 261–267.

Kuvalayananda, Swami and S. L. Vinekar. *Yoga Therapy: Its Basic Principles and Methods*. New Delhi: Ministry of Health, 1963.

Lad, Vasant, *Āyurveda: The Science of Self-Healing*. Santa Fe, New Mexico: Lotus Press, 1985.

———. *Lectures on Āyurveda* (audio cassette series, 6 vols.) Albuquerque, New Mexico: The Āyurvedic Institute, no date.

LaFleur, William R. "Saigyō and the Buddhist Value of Nature," in *Nature in*

Asian Traditions of Thought, Essays in Environmental Philosophy. Edited by J. Baird Callicott and Roger T. Ames, 183–209. Albany: State University of New York Press, 1989.

Larson, Gerald James. *Classical Sāṃkhya, An Interpretation of Its History and Meaning*. Delhi: Motilal Banarsidass, 1969, 1979.

———. "Life Sciences (Āyurveda) Old and New: In Search of New Agendas for Healing." Paper presented at the University of Hawaii Center for South Asian Studies 10th Spring Symposium: *Healing Systems of South Asia*. Honolulu, April 12, 1993.

———. "Āyurveda and the Hindu Philosophical Systems." In *Self as Body in Asian Theory and Practice*, ed. Kasulis et al., 103–21. First published in *Philosophy East and West* 37 (3) (July 1987).

Leder, Drew. *The Absent Body*. Chicago and London: University of Chicago Press, 1990.

Lee, Riley. Lecture and Performance on the *shakuhachi* flute. East-West Center. Honolulu, Hawaii, October 1993.

Levin, David Michael and George F. Soloman. "The Discursive Formation of the Body in the History of Medicine." *Journal of Medicine and Philosophy* 15 (1990) 515–37.

Locke, Kevin (Tokeya Inajin). Interviewed in *The Spirit World* [Series: *The American Indians*]. Alexandria, Virginia: Time-Life Books, 1992.

Maslow, Abraham and Bela Mittelmann. "The Meaning of 'Healthy' ('Normal') and of 'Sick' ('Abnormal')." In *Concepts of Health and Disease*, ed. Caplan, et al., 47–56.

McNeley, James K. *Holy Wind in Navajo Philosophy*. Tucson: University of Arizona Press, 1981.

Merleau-Ponty, Maurice. *Phenomenology of Perception*, trans. Colin Smith. London: Routledge and Kegan Paul, 1962.

Mishra, Kamalakar. *Significance of The Tantric Tradition*. Varanasi: Arddhanarisvara Publications, 1981.

Morais, Vamberto. "The Contribution of Yoga to Modern Life." In *The Nature of Religious Man*, edited by D. B. Fry, 119–41. London: Octagon Press, 1982.

Moses, Johnny (*Whisstemenee:* Walking Medicine Robe). SiSíWiss Medicine Teachings, First Unitarian Church of Honolulu. Honolulu, Hawaii, May 1993.

———. "Northwest Coast Medicine Teachings: An Interview with Johnny Moses," by Timothy White. *Shaman's Drum* (Spring 1991) 36–43. *See* http://johnnymoses.com

———. "Native Northwest Coast Song and Drum," Lecture/presentation at Southern Illinois University, Edwardsville, Illinois, June 14, 1996.

Nietzsche, Friedrich. *The Gay Science* [1882], trans. Walter Kaufmann. New York: Random House, 1974.

———. *The Will to Power* [1901], trans. Walter Kaufmann and R. J. Hollingdale. New York: Vintage Books, 1967.

———. *Thus Spake Zarathustra* [1892], trans. R. J. Hollingdale. Baltimore, Maryland: Penguin Books, 1977.

Numbers, Ronald L. and Darrel W. Amundsen. *Caring and Curing: Health and Medicine in the Western Religious Traditions*. New York: Macmillan, 1986.

Obenchain, Diane B. "Spiritual Quests of Twentieth-Century Women: A Theory of Self-Discovery and a Japanese Case Study." In *Self as Person in Asian Theory and Practice*, edited by Roger T. Ames, Thomas P. Kasulis, and Wimal Dissanayake, 125–168. Albany: State University of New York Press, 1993.

Organ, Troy Wilson. *The Self in Indian Philosophy*. London and the Hague: Mouton & Co., 1964.

Pandit, M. P. *Lights on the Tantra*. Madras: Ganesh and Co., 1977.

Paramananda, Swami. *Spiritual Healing*. Cohassett, Maine: Vedanta Centre Publishers, 1974, 1985.

Plato, *Collected Dialogues of Plato*, edited by Edith Hamilton and Huntington Cairns. Princeton, New Jersey: Princeton University Press, 1961.

Podgorski, Frank. "Sāṃkhya-Yoga Meditation: Psycho-Spiritual Transvaluation." *Journal of Dharma* 2 (April 1978) 152–63.

Pörn, Ingmar. "An Equilibrium Model of Health," *Health, Disease, and Causal Explanation in Medicine*, edited by L. Nordenfelt and B. I. B. Lindahl, 3–13. Dordrecht and Boston: D. Reidel, 1984.

Powers, William K. *Sacred Language: The Nature of Supernatural Discourse in Lakota*. Norman: University of Oklahoma Press, 1986.

Ramakrishnananda, Swami. Lecture: "Yoga," *Brahmavadin 1895–1914*, vol. 2: *Yoga* (1984) 1–12.

Rao, S. K. Ramachandra. *Śrī Cakra: Its Yantra, Mantra, and Tantra*. Bangalore: Kalpatharu Research Academy, 1982.

Ravindra, R. "Is Religion Psychotherapy?" *Religious Studies* 14 (Spring 1978) 389–97.

Rowell, Lewis. *Music and Musical Thought in Early India*. Chicago: University of Chicago Press, 1992.

Sanford, John A. *Healing and Wholeness*. New York: Paulist Press, 1967.

Shah, Pragna R. *Tantra: Its Therapeutic Aspect*. Calcutta: Punthi Pustak, 1987.

Sheets-Johnstone, Maxine, ed. *Giving the Body Its Due*, 132–58. Albany: State University of New York Press, 1992.

———. "The Materialization of the Body: A History of Western Medicine, A History in Process." In *Giving the Body Its Due*, 132–58.

Sheikh, Anees A. and Katherina S. Sheikh. *Eastern and Western Approaches to Healing: Ancient Wisdom and Modern Knowledge*. New York: John Wiley and Sons, 1989.

Singh, Lalan Prasad. *Tantra, Its Mystic and Scientific Basis*. Delhi: Concept Publishing Co., 1976.

Sinha, Hirendra Nath. "Dhyāna," "Prāṇāyāma," "Pratyāhāra," "Samādhi." In *Brahmavadin 1895–1914*, Vol. 2, *Yoga*, 1984.

Śivananda Yoga Vedanta Center. *The Śivananda Companion to Yoga*. New York: Simon and Schuster, 1983.

Smith, Huston, quoted in "Chant," National Public Radio Program, 1983. Honolulu: University of Hawaii Sinclair Library, audio cassette Vol. 975, 1983.

Sobel, David S. *Ways of Health, Holistic Approaches to Ancient and Contemporary Medicine*. New York and London: Harcourt Brace Jovanovich, 1979.

Sontag, Susan, *Illness as Metaphor*. New York: Vintage Books, Random House, 1977, 1979.

Staal, Frits. "Indian Bodies." In *Self as Body*, ed. Kasulis et al., 59–102.
Sullivan, Lawrence E. *Healing and Restoring: Health and Medicine in the World's Religious Traditions*. New York: Macmillan, 1989.
———. "Healing." In *The Encyclopedia of Religion*, 16 vols. Edited by Mircea Eliade, 6:226–34. New York: Macmillan, 1987.
Susser, Mervyn. "Ethical Components in the Definition of Health." In *Concepts of Health and Disease*, ed. Caplan et al., 93–105.
Tabor, Daniel C. "Ripe and Unripe: Concepts of Health and Sickness in Ayurvedic Medicine, *Social Science and Medicine* 15B (1981): 429–55.
Tillich, Paul. "The Meaning of Health." In *Religion and Medicine: Essays on Meaning, Values, and Health*, edited by David Belgum, 3–12. Ames: The Iowa State University Press, 1967.
Upadhyaya, Kashi Nath. *Early Buddhism and the Bhagavadgītā*. Delhi: Motilal Banarsidass, 1971, 1983.
Veith, Ilza, trans. *Huang Ti Nei Ching Su Wên: The Yellow Emperor's Classic of Internal Medicine*. Berkeley: University of California Press, 1949, 1972.
Virchow, Rudolph, "Three Selections from Rudolph Virchow," trans. S. G. M. Engelhardt. In *Concepts of Health and Disease*, ed. Caplan et al., 187–96.
Vivekananda, Swami. *Complete Works*, 8 vols. Calcutta: Advaita Ashrama, 1947, 1986.
Watson, Burton, trans. *The Complete Works of Chuang Tzu*. New York: Columbia University Press, 1968.
Wezler, A. "On the Quadruple Division of the Yogaśāstra, the Caturvyūhatva of the Cikitsāśāstra and the 'Four Noble Truths' of the Buddha." *Indologica Taurinensia* 12 (1984), 290–337.
Wheeler, David L. "A Physician-Anthropologist Examines What Ails America's Medical System," *Chronicle of Higher Education* 39 (39) June 2, 1993, A6–7.
Whitbeck, Caroline. "A Theory of Health." In *Concepts of Health and Disease*, ed. Caplan et al., 611–26.
Woodroffe, Sir John (Arthur Avalon). *The Garland of Letters (Varṇamālā): Studies in the Mantraśāstra*. Madras: Ganesh and Co., 1922, 1994.
———. *Introduction to Tantra Shastra*. Madras: Ganesh and Co., 1913, 1952.
World Health Organization, "Constitution of the World Health Organization." In *Concepts of Health and Disease*, ed. Caplan et al., 83–84.
Zimmer, Heinrich. *Philosophies of India*. New York: Pantheon Press [Bollingen Series Vol. 26] 1951.
Zimmermann, Francis. *The Jungle and the Aroma of Meats: An Ecological Theme in Hindu Medicine*. Berkeley: University of California Press, 1987. First published as *La Jungle et le Fumet des Viandes* by Editions du Seuil, 1982.
Zysk, Kenneth. *Asceticism and Healing in Ancient India: Medicine in the Buddhist Monastery*. New York and Oxford: Oxford University Press, 1991.
———. "Mantra in Āyurveda" in *Understanding Mantras*, edited by Harvey P. Alper. Albany: State University of New York Press, 1989.

Subject Index

Adaptation, 54–56, 76–77
Aesthetic therapeutics
  meaning of term, 140
  in Tantra, 153–57
Aesthetic(s), 7–8, 153, 157
Afflictions. *See Sanskrit terms index* Kleśa-s
Alcohol and drugs, 63, 109. *See also* Smoking
Alleviation therapy, 61
Ambiguity, 48–49, 55, 61, 62
American Indian Traditions, 9, 70
  community in, 169, 170
  curing songs, 157, 160–61
  Lakota, 161–62, 165, 170, 171–72
  Navajo, 1, 157, 160
  Samish, 160–61
  SiSí Wiss, 160–61
American Sanskrit Institute, 155
Anatomy, 18–19, 44. *See also* Physiology
Anglo-European worldview, 4–5, 6, 12, 13, 22, 158
Animals
  and dualism, 14
  human being as preeminent animal, 24–25
  in food chain, 60
  in reincarnation, 22
Art, 75, 153, 157. *See also* Aesthetic(s)
Awareness, 62–63, 66–69, 116
Āyurveda
  and yoga, 36–37, 42
  concepts of body, 36–44
  concepts of person, 7, 40, 42–44
  determinants of health, 7, 9, 46–47, 47–78, 50, 82, 134
  eight branches of medicine (table), 37
  four branches of medical knowledge (table), 46
  meaning of term, 36, 51
  medical therapeutics, 7, 167
  philosophical roots, 37, 42
  religious therapeutics, 78–82
  therapies, 56, 61

Behavioral medicine, 20
Body
  alienation from, 66
  Anglo-European views of, 11–12, 13, 17–21
  as achievement concept, 13, 116
  as instrument of sacred music, 161–62
  as repository of spiritual and healing knowledge and practices, 161, 173
  concepts and models
    as an instance of creation, 28
    as causal network, 20
    as communicative field, 20
    as conscious, 22, 72
    as container, 12–13
    as discursive formation, 19–20
    as enlightenable, 7, 153
    as instrument of enlightenment, 7, 153

Laya, 93, 147
Mantra, 93, 149–53, 155
non-Hindu, 91–92
Pūrna (Integral), 93–94
Ṣaḍaṅga, 88
Tāntric, 90, 93, 140–53
Yoga, Classical. *See also Sanskrit terms index* Yoga
as a religious therapeutic, 94–131
as a religious therapeutic (table), 84
Yoga-bhāsya, therapeutic paradigm (table), 132
Yoga-sūtras, therapeutic paradigm (table), 134
Yoking, 85-86, 135

Zen. *See* Buddhism

Sanskrit Terms

Abhāva (analytic absence), 71
Abhyāsa (persistent effort), 98, 106, 147
Ādhibhautika (sociality), 71
Adhikāra (qualification), 22
Agni (fire), 61, 169
Ahaṃkara (ego), 101, 147
Ahiṁsā (non-injury), 92. *See under* Yama-s
Āma (product of incomplete digestion), 60–61
Āmaya (sickness), 109
Ananta (the infinite), 114
Antaraṅga and bahiraṅga (inner and outer limbs of Yoga), 123
Antarāyāḥ (obstacles), 103–4
  nine obstacles (list), 103
Anuloma Viloma (alternate nostril breathing), 119–20
Anunāsika (nasalizing script-mark), 151
Anusvāra (nasalizing script-mark), 151
Ārogya (health), 65, 109, 133
Āsana-s (postures). *See under* Yoga
Ātman (Self), 21
  in *Upaniṣads*, 25–26, 171
  in Vedānta, 3
  in *Vedas*, 23, 88
Ātma-pratyabhijña (self-knowledge), 34
Aum. *See* Om
Avidyā (the affliction of ignorance). *See under* kleśa-s
  as a cognitive disease, 101
Bandha ('lock' of energy), 148
Bhavaroga (disease of rebirth and suffering), 110
Bhavavyādhi (ills of existence), 154
Bhoga (enjoyment), 145, 146
Bhukti vs. *mukti* (worldly enjoyment vs. liberation), 146
Bīja-s, *Bīja-mantra-s* (seed sounds), 150–53, 188n47
  and cakras, 148
Bindu (drop, dot)
  in Śri Yantra, 143
Brahman (the One that is All)
  in Āyurveda, 63
  in Sāṃkhya, 28
  in Tantra, 29, 32–33, 88, 150, 156, 161
  in *Upaniṣads*, 25, 88, 171
  in Vedānta, 32
  in *Vedas*, 24
Buddhi (intelligence; faculty of discriminative knowing), 88, 95, 97, 99–100, 101–2, 108–9, 147
  as first evolute of *prakṛti*, 99–100

Cakra-s ('wheels'; centers of energy), 92, 142, 144, 146–49, 150–51, 187n13
  seven cakras (table), 148
Candrabindu ('dot in a moon' [= *anunāsika*]), 151
Citta (thirteen-part instrument of cognition: *ahaṃkara, buddhi, manas*, five senses, and five organs of action), 101–2

Index of Names

Sanskrit Texts